Contents

KW-054-045

Acknowledgements

Thanks to the International Planned Parenthood Federation for the use of their excellent library.

Thanks to the Institute of Child Health at the University of London for their friendly support and for the use of their resources, including illustrations. Special thanks to Professor David Morley for his encouragement and advice.

Thanks to Sister Pauline Dean for her advice on Chapter 1, based on her work in West Africa with young women.

Thanks to the London International Group, plc, manufacturers of Durex, and to The Nuffield Foundation for their generous financial support which will enable this book to be available at a considerably reduced price.

Thanks to the students of St Augustine's School, Zimbabwe who through our lessons, discussion and friendship, taught me what they wanted to learn about themselves and their relationships. Special thanks to Gibson Bhunu for his helpful comments on the manuscript.

Thanks to John Guillebaud, Medical Director of the Margaret Pyke Centre for Training in Family Planning, and author of *The Pill*, for his expert advice on the manuscript.

Thanks to the Centre for African Family Studies, Nairobi, for advice and criticism, and to Stephanie Kinyanjui for helpful, encouraging comments on the manuscript.

Thanks to Alan Thomas for taking the photographs. Cover photograph courtesy of Juliet Highet.

Thanks to TALC for the illustrations on pages 75 and 76.

Foreword

by Fred T. Sai

It is both a privilege and a pleasure to be asked to write the fore-word to this excellent guide to sexual relationships, in which physical development and reproduction are placed within the context of the emotional maturity and adult qualities so necessary to marriage and parenthood. Although increasingly 'family health', and 'population education' are being introduced into school curricula in African countries, very few programmes directly address reproductive biology, and the practical knowledge necessary for sexual activity to take place in an atmosphere of mutual respect and trust. I hope that this book will be used widely, not only by the relatively few enrolled in secondary schools and colleges, but by youth groups of all types, and by parents. Too many young people grow up uninformed. Too many adults do not know how to discuss these delicate issues with their children.

Janie Hampton addresses this book to the adolescents now, or soon to be, facing the physical changes, feelings and decisions involved in healthy living and healthy loving. However, perhaps in this foreword I may be permitted to set this endeavour in the context of what is currently known about the reproductive life and health of young people in Africa, a context in which the need for a book such as this becomes plain.

In most African countries south of the Sahara more than half of all women get married in their teenage years and have a baby soon after. The risks of pregnancy and childbirth to these mothers are higher than to mothers aged 20 to 30, and so are the risks to their babies. Some of these risks may be due, especially at very young ages, under 16, to the incomplete physical development of the mother. Others are due to the lifestyle, or the social situation typical of many adolescents, which reduces the chance that they will seek out, or get, good antenatal and postnatal care. If this book increases awareness of the responsibility young mothers and fathers bear to themselves and their children, to have their children when they are biologically, socially and psychologically ready for them, and the importance of good health care, then it will have served an invaluable purpose.

Youngsters who do not marry in their teenage years, however, may also engage in sexual activity. Some surveys have shown that only a few unmarried women have not had sexual intercourse by the time they are 21, while almost half the single young women aged 17 and under have had sexual experience. The number of induced abortions is growing among young women, especially the unmarried, and since in most African countries abortion is illegal, it carries great risks to life, health and future fertility. Although the use of contraception by unmarried women, particularly those in secondary and higher education, is higher than average, still less than half the young women at risk of pregnancy are current users.

Another great risk to health and future fertility attendant upon early and uninformed sexual activity is that of sexually transmitted disease. Somewhere between 15 and 30 percent of young people aged 15 to 24 may already have contracted such a disease. The consequences for future fertility, of untreated gonorrhoea and chlamydia, are grave. In parts of Central and West Africa 21 to 40 percent of women remain childless at the end of their childbearing years — and STD is indicated as one of the prime causes.

This book was probably written before the full enormity of the AIDS epidemic was apparent, making Mrs. Hampton's advice even more important.

Information and education on sexuality and reproduction are vital if young people are to behave responsibly. Society, too, has an obligation to set consistent standards and to provide individuals with the means to act responsibly. It is inconsistent to permit marriage at very young ages and then expect the young people still in school to refrain from sexual activity. There must also be wide access to health care. Family planning services in particular must be freely available to all, not only to men, or to married women, or to people over a certain age. Universal counselling on socially acceptable behaviour including the ability to say no to pressures to engage in early sex should be part of all types of education.

Individual knowledge and understanding, supported by information and services, is the best way to secure healthy living. I wholeheartedly commend this book to teachers, health workers, youth workers and parents, and to all who have responsibility for the education and health of young people.

Introduction

Family life education is being taught in more and more schools and colleges. But there are still many young people who have no idea how their bodies work, how pregnancy happens, or how to prevent unwanted pregnancies. Many of the readers of this book are not yet sexually active. This book is not meant to encourage them to experiment with sex. They may be thinking, 'I don't need to know about contraception or sexually transmitted diseases'. They may not plan to get married for many years. I hope they will read these chapters anyway. Then they will know where to find the information when they do become sexually active. The information is important *before* anyone embarks on sexual activity. An unwanted pregnancy can happen the very first time that a person has sex. Several studies of young people have shown that those who have been taught about reproduction, relationships and contraception are *less* likely to have irresponsible sexual relationships.

Deciding to have sex with someone is a big decision, usually occurring at marriage. Anyone who wants sex before marriage should think carefully about it first and make sure there is no risk of becoming pregnant, catching a disease, hurting their partner's feelings or ruining their life while still at school.

The last chapter in the book is included to complete the guide to healthy living. There are many pressures on young people nowadays to eat expensive processed foods with no nutrition, to take illegal and dangerous drugs, to smoke cigarettes and to drink too much alcohol. Few young people understand the dangers of these things – they only see the glamorous image projected by advertisments.

If this book prevents just one unwanted pregnancy, or one accident from alcohol; if it stops one person from smoking, one person from passing on an STD, or one person from trying out drugs, then all the hard work will have been worthwhile.

I would be pleased to receive any comments or suggestions from readers.

Notes to teachers

Discussions

Many topics in this book may be easier to understand after a group discussion. Some young people find it easier to talk about sexuality if there are no adults around. Others may want help and guidance.

When planning a discussion the leader should prepare the subject well so that questions can be answered correctly. If the leader does not know the answer, then be honest and suggest ways of finding the answer. Never try and reject a question or topic because the answer is unknown or it is embarrassing. Young people want to talk about everything, especially taboo subjects. They need to understand why the subject is taboo and how this relates to their lives.

Language should be kept simple and informal, using words that everybody understands.

Young people may be embarrassed to ask the questions they really want to. Ask everyone in the group to write their questions on a piece of paper. The leader can then try and answer the question without any embarrassment to anyone.

Leaders should try not to impose their values and personal opinions on the group, but discover what everyone present thinks. Try not to judge different beliefs or ideas. Young people are surrounded by different values from newspapers, parents, television, films, teachers. Part of growing up is sorting out which of these values they want to live by. Discussing different topics can help young people to sort out the conflicting values of modern society.

Keep the discussion light. Although all the subjects covered in *Healthy Living, Healthy Loving* are serious, they can be treated with a sense of humour!

Some subjects may need an 'expert' to lead the discussion and share their knowledge. For example, a lesson on pregnancy would be good if the local midwife were present and could share her knowledge with the class.

More than 12 in a group affects the involvement of everyone: some members may feel too shy to speak. If the group is large, then divide it into several smaller groups of five or six people.

The arrangement of seating has an effect on discussions too. Sitting in straight rows with the leader at the front stifles the sharing of ideas. Sitting in a circle so that everybody can see everybody else makes everyone feel involved and want to participate. The person who says the most may not have the best ideas. Encourage everyone to join in.

Role-play

Role-play is an effective way of learning and teaching combined. Children learn about parenthood through their games of 'mother and father'.

Young people can use role-play to act out situations that they may later find themselves in. All types of experiences can be explored, without the problems of the real situations. Role-play does not need a script or the learning of lines. The players simply discuss the subject for a few minutes and then improvise the way that kind of character would act in that situation. For example, a drunk man walking down a street, bumping into things and abusing people. Some people are better at acting than others, but everyone should be given a chance to join in. The play need only last a few minutes.

After a role-play the players and the group discuss the topic and what they learnt from the play. The role-play should be used to bring out problems relating to the subject under discussion. For example, the consequences of pre-marital sex, cigarette smoking or getting drunk.

CHAPTER 1
Relationships

Growing up

Growing up starts when we learn to express our own ideas. It means learning how to cope with the world without the protection and help of our parents. Independent and mature people are able to control their actions and feelings. They can think clearly. They can understand and respect how other people think and feel. A mature person is unselfish.

Maturity does not come to us easily. We all have to learn by our mistakes. But *physical* maturity — the way our body grows up — is something outside our control. Between the ages of eleven and eighteen, changes happen which make it possible for us to become parents. The child's body turns into an adult's body. The problem that many teenagers face is that the maturity of their thoughts and feelings may not be able to keep pace with the maturity of their bodies. They want to 'make love' before they have any real love to give. They are not old enough to cope with the responsibilities that making love brings, such as pregnancy and long term relationships.

There is no easy answer to this problem. No book can tell you how to recognise true love or how to choose your life partner. But it is helpful to talk about it with friends and to know what is happening to us. If we can understand the changes, then it is easier to accept them. Knowledge helps us to become mature.

Loving is giving, not giving so that we can get something nice back, just plain giving. Many people want love because they cannot love their own selves. They find it hard to give back love in return, so their relationships turn sour. Mature people are not perfect. But they have learnt to accept themselves. Only then do they find the strength to give unconditionally.

Loving is receiving, not receiving because we feel we have deserved it, just plain receiving. It is often harder to receive than to give because it makes us open to being wounded. It is safer to receive love from a mature person because they are trustworthy. They do not need to despise other people who are disabled or poor or belong to a different tribe or religion. Nor do they love people just because they are handsome or pretty.

When we are mature, we have confidence. We can overcome

fears and difficulties. We do not blame other people. Life is often unfair and everyone has problems. Some people may find school work difficult; some people may feel they are not very beautiful or strong; some people may have difficulty getting on with their parents. We can all overcome our difficulties with patience, work and the love of our friends.

It is sensible to ask for help and advice and to support your friends when they are in need. The greatest gift in life (much more lasting than sexual love!) is friendship between people.

Friendship

Friendship is a close relationship where sexual attraction is not felt. Teenagers are usually friends with a person of the same age and sex or with a brother or sister. Older people may make more varied friends. Friendship is a kind of love and it is very valuable and important. Friends enjoy being with each other, laughing, talking and sharing possessions. They also share secrets. Friends can trust each other. Close friends are people who will always help and support you because they are fond of you and like to receive your affection. Not everyone we meet can become a close friend. There may be only a few in your whole life. Finding a new friend need not make your other friends jealous. There are different things to like in each person and different things to talk about and do. Often a group of friends like to go around together. A happy gang of friends will give equally and share ideas. A bullying leader is not a real friend.

> Friendship is unselfish love that gives and receives freely.

Sexual attraction

Children learn about friendship. But sexual attraction is a new experience which happens when our bodies begin to change into adult ones (see Chapter 2 page 13). Sexual attraction is a strong feeling which is hard to control, like being very hungry or thirsty or tired. A hungry person desires food and the first mouthful is a great pleasure. In the same way teenage girls and boys want to hug and kiss each other. As they grow older, they may want to have sexual intercourse with each other. There is nothing wrong in these desires. They are a natural result of our bodies changing. Are we angry with a man who is hungry? It would be pointless because hunger can happen to us all. The same is true of sexual attraction.

However, wanting to have sex is not quite the same as hunger. There are three reasons for this.

1 Sex takes place between *two* people. So the desire in the body

2

also involves a relationship with another person.

2   The result of making love is that the woman can become pregnant and have a baby.

3   Because sex is a new desire, and a very strong and pleasurable one, it is easy to become greedy for it.

Let us discuss these reasons for being careful about sex.

1   Both men and women can easily be attracted to someone who does not return the feeling. When this happens, the man may be tempted to force himself on the woman. Or the woman may try to seduce the man by showing off her breasts or flashing her eyes at him. Such men and women may have many sexual partners. Their happiness lasts for a few moments before and during the sex act. But afterwards they feel miserable. The man may be arrested and sent to prison for rape. The woman may get pregnant. Either partner may catch a dangerous disease (see Chapter 6). This is not 'making love'! Sexual attraction on its own is not enough to bring real lasting happiness. A man cannot enjoy his power if he uses it without respect for his sex partner. Such a man has lost his honour and he will grow to hate himself. Some men pay money to prostitutes for easy sex. Love cannot be bought and sold. Both the man and the woman are destroying a wonderful gift.

2   The feelings of sexual desire are intended to produce babies. The desire is a strong, natural force. It makes sure that our families will continue into the future. Being a parent means being emotionally and mentally and spiritually mature. The way to prevent unwanted babies is described in Chapter 5. The best way for teenagers to prevent pregnancy is to say 'No'. Teenagers must make sure they do not get into situations where saying 'No' is difficult.

3   Sexual desire is a new experience for the teenager. It is very exciting and many thoughts and conversations will be about sex. But like all desires, it can easily become boring or even revolting if we allow it to grow too large. Imagine how boring it would be to listen to someone talking about nothing but food for months and months! Imagine how revolting it would be to eat and eat until you are sick! Sexual desire can be like this too, even if you do not realise it at first. We enjoy it more if we can resist the temptation to be greedy.

What is sexual pleasure?

Many people think that sex means having intercourse. But this is only a part of sexual pleasure. All over our bodies there are places called **erogenous zones** where sexual pleasure lies in wait. In each person these can be different. Your lover may like to have her ears or her fingers or her toes sucked or kissed. You may like to have your back rubbed or tickled or scratched lightly with the fingernails. It is possible to enjoy each other's bodies without having intercourse. But first you have to talk to each other and agree about this and be content. Then the pleasure you share will be 'making love'. Intercourse is a very important experience. It is the moment when two bodies and two souls can be joined.

The body is the home of our soul. Treat it with care.

Falling in love

Falling in love is a wonderful and powerful experience which is beyond our control. It includes friendship and sexual attraction. But there is something more as well. Lovers worship each other. They are blind to each other's faults. They can do little else except think and dream about each other. Their happiness spreads outwards. Even the dullest day becomes bright when you are in love. We call this 'romance'. A romantic world is a perfect one where nothing can go wrong.

Falling in love can happen several times in a lifetime and it can happen in different ways. Young people may fall in love often. This can be very passionate but it may not last long. After a few weeks or months, or even a year or two, two people can grow apart because they each want something different out of life. Young people are still changing and building their personalities.

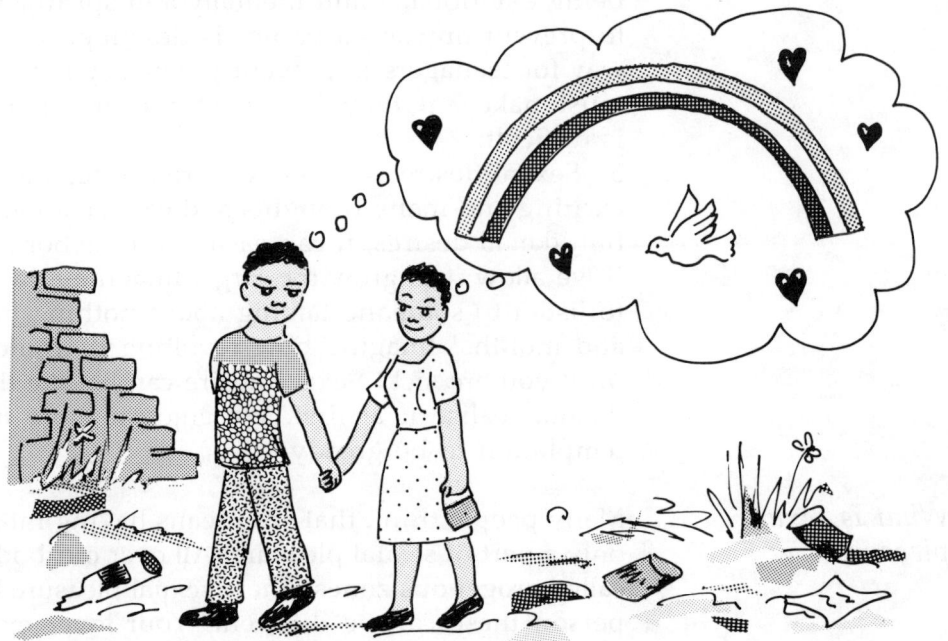

The world feels like a beautiful place when you are in love.

4

Their relationships are like experiments. They are learning how to love. Learning the difference between love and **lust** is part of growing up.

The most difficult lesson is not how to *give* love. Sexual attraction usually takes care of that! It is how to *receive* love. We can only take love from other people when we feel we deserve it. This means being emotionally and spiritually mature. Until we know and understand and accept ourselves, the two-way relationship of love will be difficult. We may become selfish, or jealous or over-emotional.

> To be loved, we must respect ourselves.

Myth: Love lives in my heart and so when my heart beats faster at someone, I must be in love with him.

Truth: Love is not just in the heart. But sexual attraction makes the blood run faster through our veins. Do not confuse sexual desire with love.

Myth: Women like powerful, dominating men who tell them what to do.

Truth: Power is only attractive when it is used with respect and consideration. It is ugly and brutal when it is used selfishly. Women like men who care about them, as people with feelings.

Myth: Sexual desire is caused by women and it is their fault if they get pregnant.

Truth: Sexual attraction is caused by chemicals called hormones in the bodies of men and women. A man always shares equal responsibility for a pregnancy.

Myth: Women often say 'no' to encourage a man to get excited. What they really mean is 'yes'.

Truth: Men can easily imagine that what they want is also what the woman wants. Because of the strength of their desire, they can easily deceive themselves.

No woman should ever be *persuaded* to have sex, in any way at all.

Myth: 'They fell in love and lived happily ever after.'
Truth: The real world is not a romantic place. To last until death, a love affair needs tender care, like a young plant!

5

Dear Auntie,

I am a 19 year old school girl. I believe in Women's Liberation. My boy-friend says he loves me very much and when we leave school we will get married. But whenever we meet, he always thinks of sex. He forces me until at last he does it. I never expected him to do such a thing. I don't feel free in any way. Do you think he really loves me?

Blessing

Dear Blessing,

Your boyfriend is using you to satisfy his sexual desire. If he really loved you, then he would wait until you left school and get married to him. He would never force himself on you. Having sex with a man because he insists is not making love. Freedom or liberation for women does not mean that women should have sex before marriage. Liberation means women making their own minds up, and having the freedom to say 'No'.

No-one should feel that they must have sex with their partners. There are several phrases that men say to women in order to encourage them to have sex.

For example, 'All the other girls do', 'You are only a child if you don't', 'I will only love you if you do', or 'You cannot get pregnant the first time'. None of these are true. Men often say 'Don't worry, I'll marry you' — and then they disappear when the girl gets pregnant.

Be strong with your boyfriend. Tell him to wait until you get married. If he cannot wait, then tell him you are not interested in him any more.

Marriage

There are many reasons why people get married. It may be arranged by their parents. It may be because the woman is pregnant. It may be through fear of loneliness. It may be for the sake of a land settlement or money. It may be because they have fallen in love. Getting married is a very big decision and one of the most important events in a person's life. It is the beginning of a new life shared with another person. The real question is how do we make a good, loving, lasting marriage?

For a good marriage, a couple need friendship, love and sexual attraction. They need to be mature adults, able to give and to receive love. In a good marriage, the partners share a promise not to love anyone else. This promise is freely given by both of them. It cannot mean that the man owns the woman, or that the woman owns the man.

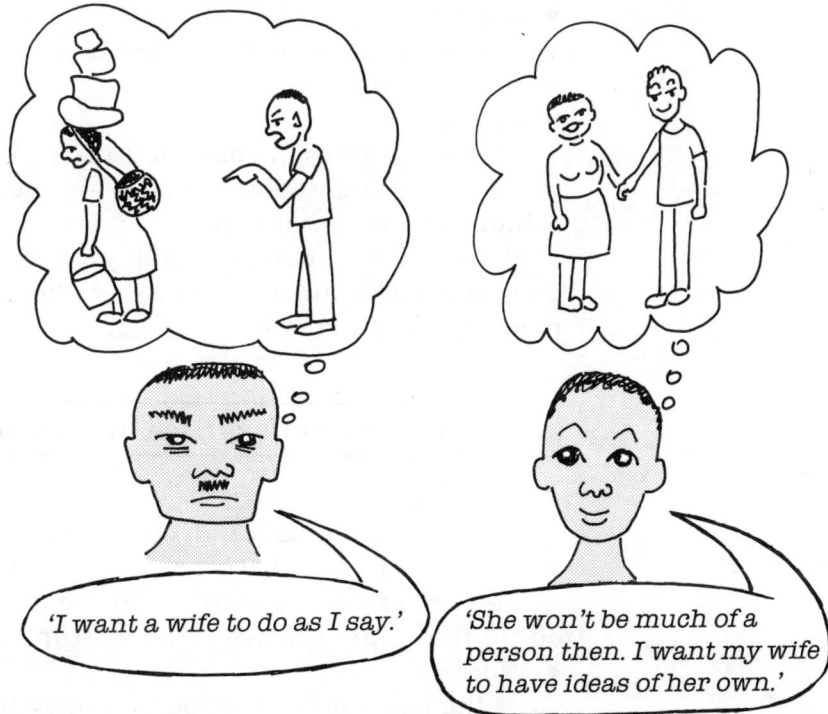

'I want a wife to do as I say.'

'She won't be much of a person then. I want my wife to have ideas of her own.'

What do you think a wife should be?

True marriage is not ownership but a shared promise to belong to one another.

In every country women make up half the population. And often, their hard work produces more than half their country's wealth. But women are often thought to be incapable of making their own decisions as mature adults. Men who believe this are marrying a woman who is a work-animal, like a donkey. Which would you rather marry? A donkey woman who brays and kicks because she is unhappy, or a beautiful and loving woman who is proud to be your wife?

A good marriage is a union of four things.

● The heart

The couple feel joy and contentment in being together. They like to make each other happy and think of special ways to do this. They share their sorrows too.

● The mind

They feel naturally at ease with each other and often read each other's thoughts. They help each other to learn. They are modest and unselfish and patient with each other. They discuss everything important, respecting each other's opinions.

- The soul

They live truthfully with one another. They have the same vision for their future.

- The body

The husband gives his body to satisfy his wife and the wife gives herself to bring satisfaction to her husband. By giving, both achieve a deeper happiness.

Marriage helps two people to grow close to one another but it does not make them the same. Rather it gives them the confidence to be different!

> In the unity of marriage, we can enjoy our diversity.

There are also practical decisions which a couple must make. It is best to discuss these *before* you get married. It will show whether the romance of love and the attraction of sex is supported by the commonsense of friendship!

- Work

Does the husband earn enough money from his work to support his wife and his family? Does the wife also have a job? Does her husband believe his wife should work for money? Is there someone to work in the fields, prepare the meals and clean the house? If this is the wife's job, does her husband appreciate that it is also hard work?

- Money

Who will look after the money and who will spend it? How will they plan their spending on food, clothing, rent and furniture? How much will they save? Will they have separate accounts at the bank or building society, or a joint one?

- Housing

Will they be able to live together? Where will they live? Will they have their own house? Will they rent one or build one of their own?

- Children

Do they want to start having children as soon as they are married? Or wait for a year or two? How many children do they want? What type of contraception will they use?

- The extended family

What responsibilities do they have for other members of their families? How much of their time and money do they plan to share with their families?

- Faith

Do they share the same religious beliefs? If not, can they agree so that this difference does not affect their loving relationship? Does the difference cause problems for their families? What faith will their children be taught?

● Social life

What do they like doing when they go out together? Will they both be happy if each spends some time with other friends?

Any one of these problems, or several of them together, can be enough to cause a divorce. Discussion beforehand can save heartbreak later.

A married couple have to work together to keep their love and happiness. Many people think that when their relationship starts to fall apart, this shows they chose the wrong partner. Often couples do not realise that a relationship must develop and grow to remain loving and happy. The mother may be too busy with babies and children to think about her husband. He may be too busy with his job to think much about his wife. They live without noticing each other or thinking about their partnership. A man and wife need to spend some time together on their own, without the interruptions of the rest of the family.

When the children are older, the couple may suddenly realise that the marriage is not as good as it was. It may be too late to make the marriage good again. A failing marriage affects the children as well as the husband and wife. The children suffer from living in an unhappy home without love and without respect between the parents. Children of divorced parents may have unsuccessful marriages when they grow up.

Married people need to continue to grow and to change just like everyone else. To grow together, they need to talk openly

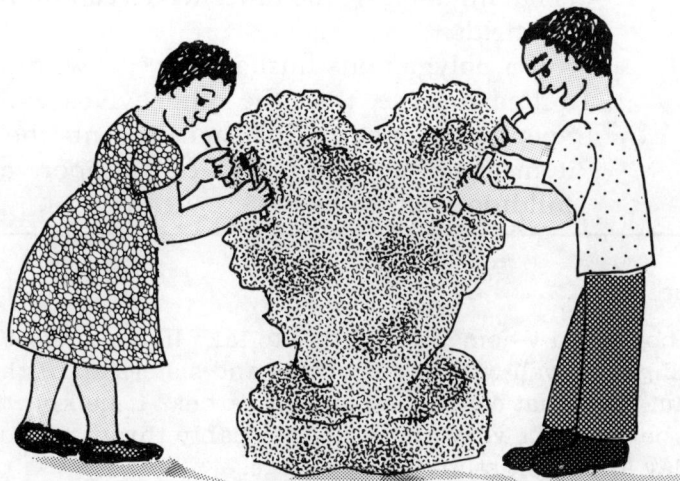

'Marriage should be a work of love', Father Motuli.

and truthfully to each other throughout their lives. Most problems can be solved by discussion if they are dealt with quickly.

If you need help with your marriage, your parents or your in — laws may not be the best people to help. They may not be able to see the problem fairly from both sides. An older married couple whom you both respect may be more helpful.

Tips for a happy marriage

- Be open and truthful. Have a regular time each week when you discuss things together.
- Treat each other fairly.
- Do not nag or criticise each other.
- Learn to apologise and to forgive each other.
- Respect and satisfy each other's sexual needs.

Polygamy

Polygamy used to be popular because a man could show he was rich enough to take extra wives. Now many men take more than one wife even when they cannot afford it. So he may have too many children to support and feed well. The husband may not treat all his wives and children equally, so they may become jealous of each other.

Polygamy has advantages to some people. Every woman has a husband, a home and children. If a husband dies, then his brother can marry the widow so she and her children are not left alone. But the widow may not like her dead husband's brother! While one wife is pregnant, the husband has another wife to sleep with. The baby can be breastfed for longer, which helps to space the children. But sexual intercourse does not harm the baby or the mother during pregnancy or breastfeeding. While one wife is having a baby, the other wives can do the work in the home or the fields.

If a polygamous husband or one wife catches a sexually transmitted disease, then the other wives will also become infected. Keeping to only one partner prevents the spread of disease, and it means that a husband can support and love his wife and children well.

Dear Auntie,

I have a boyfriend whom I would like to take home to meet my family. I am sure he will get on well with my brothers and sisters and I think my mother will like him. But what can I do about my father? If he knew that I have a boyfriend, he would be very angry and probably throw me out. He thinks I spend all day and night studying at college.

Eva

Dear Eva,

Many young women have your problem. Society is changing and parents sometimes find it is difficult to accept these changes. Fathers have always been jealous of men who are interested in their daughters. Their love for their daughters makes them very protective and unable to recognise that girls grow into women. Fathers want the best for their daughters, so your father's behaviour shows that he loves you.

Why not start by taking your boyfriend to your home together with some other friends? Don't say 'This is my boyfriend'. Introduce him as one of your friends? Then your parents will not feel threatened by the thought of a man coming to take away their daughter. They will get to know him first.

Taking boyfriends home is a good way to find out how much you really like them. Brothers and sisters can sometimes see things in a boyfriend or girlfriend that one had not noticed before. However much you love each other, marriage is partly the union of two families. If you don't like each other's family, it puts a strain on the best of marriages.

Dear Auntie,

I have been going out with a great girl for eight months and we plan to get married when we have finished college at the end of this year. We are very much in love, but my older sister says we don't really know each other.

James

Dear James,

Why do you have to think about marriage yet? Why not just enjoy each other's company first? Don't plan to get married just because you go to the cinema together, or share meals at restaurants. The longer you know each other, the better chance you have to get to know each other's strengths and weaknesses. Happy, long-lasting marriages are more often those where a couple have known each other for at least two years, if not longer. Don't rush into marriage. Spend more time learning about each other. A wedding is much easier than divorce. It is worth waiting to make sure that the rest of your life is happy and fulfilling.

Activities

1   Find out if there is a youth leadership training programme in your area. These programmes train parents, teachers, youth leaders and young people in community development; family life education; communication and personal relationships. They may be run by the Ministry of Education, or Youth, or a religious organisation.

2   Discuss the best age to get married. What qualities would you like in a husband or wife? How would you keep your marriage happy?

3   Discuss the different moral values that influence young people from parents, schools, places of worship, newspapers, magazines, books, films and television. Which values are most appropriate for a happy life and modern society?

4   Cut out letters from problems pages in newspapers and magazines. Cut off the answers, or cover them up. Discuss the problems in the letters and how the group would solve them. At the end of the discussion read the printed answer. Does the group agree with the printed answer?

5   Make a role-play about different married couples and how they treat each other. Which are the happiest marriages?

CHAPTER 2
Changing bodies

Puberty and adolescence

Puberty means the physical changes from a child, to an adult capable of becoming a parent. **Adolescence** is the years between childhood and adulthood, from the beginning of puberty to reaching the physical and emotional maturity of adulthood. This can take 10 years, between the ages of about 12 years and 20 years. Most people are mature in body, thought and responsibility by 21 years. Many people are parents and have jobs by that age.

After puberty men and woman look different. Some of the body changes are the same. Skin sweats more and acne may appear. Pubic hair grows and the face grows longer. There is a sudden growth in height. By 20 years men and woman are mature adults. The woman's breasts have grown, her hips have widened and buttocks fattened. She has monthly periods.

The man's chest and shoulders broaden and muscles get stronger, genitals grow, sperm are produced, voice deepens and hair grows on his face and chest.

By 50 years most women have reached the menopause. The ovaries make less sex hormones and menstruation stops. The skin becomes less supple and the breasts may sag. She is infertile, but enjoys making love.

A man of 65 years is fertile and can enjoy making love for the rest of his life. If they take exercise, eat well and do not smoke older people can remain fit and healthy, though bones and muscles may ache.

Apart from genitals the bodies of boys and girls look similar. A 10 year old child has learnt most skills needed for living, but needs the care and protection of the family.

The stages of growth.

13

Adolescence begins with puberty when sex **hormones** are produced in the body. Between the ages of 8 and 15 years hormones stimulate the body to mature into an adult.

Women's sex hormones are produced in the ovaries. Men's sex hormones are produced in the testicles. The hormones carry messages all over the body, causing changes and growth.

Most teenagers are excited by the adult changes in their bodies. Some teenagers may not want to accept their new bodies — the changes appear too soon. Boys may be embarrassed by their new voices, or girls feel shy about growing breasts. If children are taught what will happen at puberty, then they will understand the changes when they arrive.

The changes of puberty vary by several years. Some girls start having periods at 9 years and others start at 18 years. Periods may start within a few months, or two years of breasts growing. The average age for puberty is earlier in girls than boys. This is most obvious at about 14 years when many girls look like young women and boys have only just begun to become men. With boys the range is from 11 years to 18. Young men may continue growing in height into their early twenties.

Most people want to be like their friends. Boys who shave once a week wish they were like their friends who shave every day. Some girls try to hide their growing breasts while other girls hide their flat chests!

No-one should think it is their fault if they develop earlier or later than their friends. The average age of puberty is getting earlier as children's **nutrition** improves.

Unfortunately many adults assume that physically mature teenagers are also mentally more mature. This is not always true. A young man of 17 who shaves every day is not always more responsible than his friend who never shaves. If teenagers are treated as responsible people, then they are more likely to behave in a responsible way.

Both boys and girls are suddenly attracted and excited by the opposite sex. They begin to think more about their faces, hair and clothes.

Ideal men and women

Magazines, books and films show only 'ideal' men and women. They strengthen the idea that a woman has to have big breasts, smooth skin and a tiny waist to be normal. The 'ideal' man is tough, strong, aggressive, unemotional and never cries. He has a broad chest, tiny waist, and rippling muscles. The 'ideal' woman is weak, cannot think straight, is pretty and silly.

Every real person is different. Very few people look like the men and women in films and magazines. A woman with small breasts is just as much a woman as another woman with big

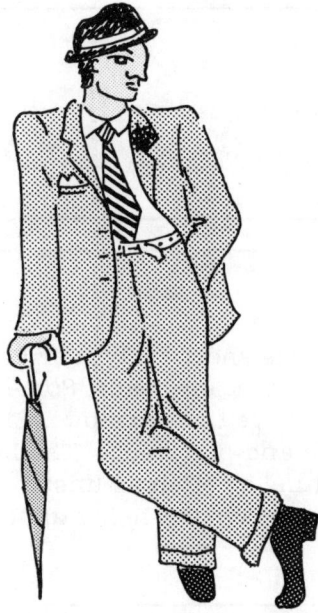

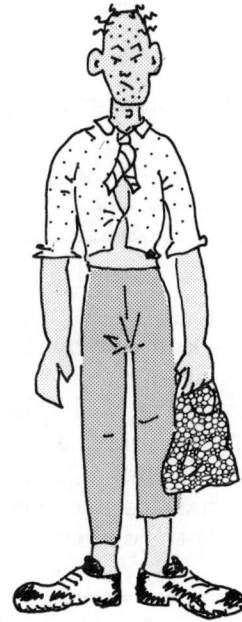

Real life and fantasy.

breasts. A man with a thick beard and hairy chest is not stronger than a man with few hairs on his chin.

Whatever anyone looks like, they can still have an attractive personality. An enormous nose, short fat legs and sticking out ears can be part of the beautiful character of a person.

The bodies of men and women are different. But apart from bearing children, men and women can do and think all the same things. There is no physical difference between the male and female brain. The difference in a man's or woman's behaviour is because of the way they are brought up. Girls are taught to like housework and child care and show their emotions. Boys are expected to be good at engineering and not to show their emotions, such as crying. In the old days all teachers were men, but nowadays many teachers are women. Women do heavy work in the fields, but many people are surprised to see women driving tractors or working as engineers.

Puberty and girls Up until puberty the bodies of girls and boys look alike. If a girl wears jeans and has short hair she looks like a boy. From around 8 years female sex hormones begin to turn a girl into a woman. She will not feel the first changes. Her uterus and vagina grow in size and her hips start to widen. Her family will notice that she grows faster in height. A 12 year old girl or boy grows as fast as a 2 year old child.

15

Dear Auntie,

Why does hair grow under the arms?

Lizzie

Dear Lizzie,

No-one knows why, but every adult has short curly hair growing in their armpits, even if they have straight hair on their heads. Some people find it very attractive, while others prefer to shave their armpits. Like beards on men's faces, this is a matter of fashion and preference. The hair soon grows back again. Shaved armpits need washing as often as unshaven armpits. If you do shave or use special cream that makes the hair fall out, be careful not to damage the delicate skin.

Breasts

The growth of breasts is the first sign to most girls that puberty has begun. The nipple grows first and is the most sensitive part of the breast. The darker area around the nipple is called the areola. The skin of the areola and the nipple is thicker than ordinary skin.

Women's breasts continue changing all through their lives. During pregnancy and breastfeeding the breasts grow to produce milk. The 15 to 20 milk ducts are protected by cushions of fat. The size and shape of the breasts depend on the amount of fat. If a woman gets fatter, then her breasts will grow.

Exercise cannot make breasts bigger, but sports such as swimming will strengthen the chest muscles which hold up the breasts. This can make them appear bigger.

The size of the breasts has no relation to how much milk they can produce or how attractive they are to men. Some men like small breasts, some men like big ones. Few men love a woman just because of the size of her breasts! Breasts are part of love-making. Feeling and sucking them is enjoyable for both the man and the woman.

Growing breasts may be uncomfortable or sore at times, especially if they rub against rough clothing, or bump into something.

If a girl feels comfortable without a bra then she need not wear one, though the weight of heavy breasts can stretch the fibres that support them. Once these fibres are stretched they cannot shrink again, so the breasts will hang down. Never buy a bra

Nipple

Areola

Milk ducts

Fat to protect breasts

Elastic fibres to support breasts

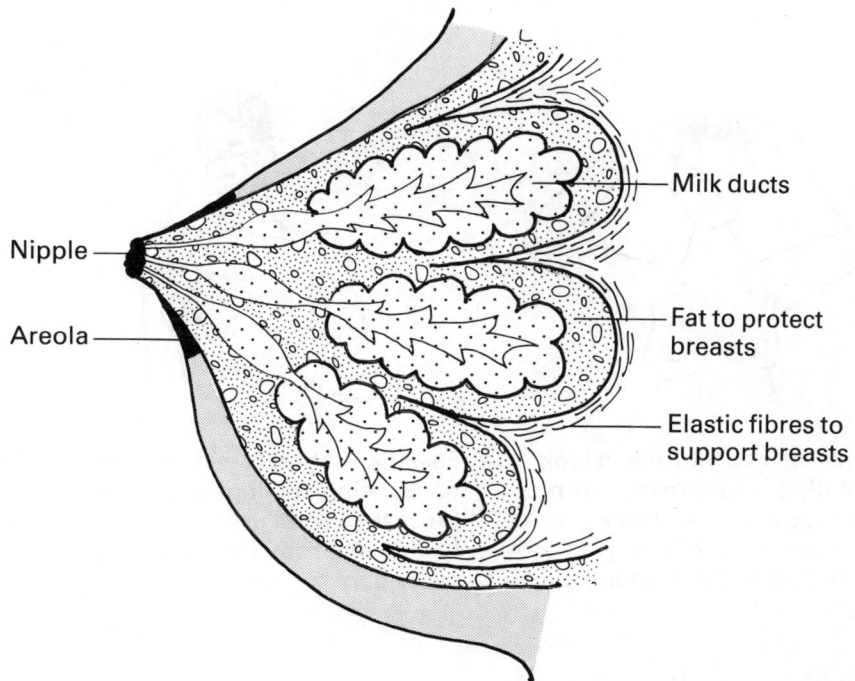

Inside the breast.

that is too small as it will cut into the back and squeeze the breasts.

The breasts of many women become swollen and tender a few days before a menstrual period. After the period they return to normal. Sometimes strange lumps appear in one or both breasts. Most lumps are harmless, but occasionally the lump is **cancer**. Breast cancer kills more women than any other type of cancer, but it can be treated if it is found early. Although breast cancer in young women is very rare, it can happen. If all young women check their breasts every month then when they are older they will recognise strange lumps.

Breast check

You know the shape and texture of your breast better than anyone else, even a doctor. So if you check your breasts every month you will notice any strange lumps.

Check after a menstrual period when the breasts are least full. Before a period the breasts may be bigger and any lumps will be difficult to feel.

Lie down on the floor or a bed. Put a pillow or a folded blanket under the right shoulder. Put the right hand behind the head. This spreads the breast evenly over the chest. Use the left hand to

17

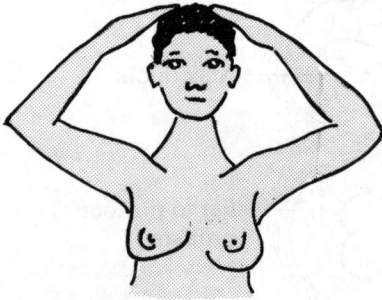

Sit in front of a mirror and look carefully at your breasts. Turn from side to side and look underneath. Look for anything unusual, especially around the nipple.

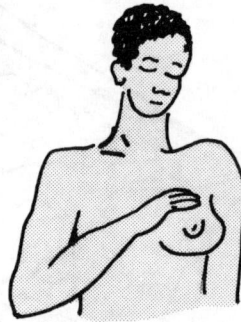

Feel the left breast with the right hand, using flat fingers together. Press the breast gently all round, feeling out from the nipple. Feel every part.

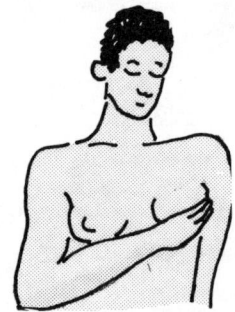

Repeat on the other breast. Be thorough and do not rush.

How to examine the breasts.

feel the right breast gently with the flat of the fingers, not the fingertips. Move the fingers in small circles all over the breasts. Repeat on the left breast with the pillow under the left shoulder. Lumps most often occur between the nipple and armpit.

If you notice any strange lump, swelling or **discharge** from the nipple then visit a health centre as soon as possible. Most breast lumps or swellings are not cancer, but all changes should be checked. If left alone, breast cancer will not get better — it will spread to other parts of the body.

Look out for:
- Strange lumps, large or small.
- Unusual changes in the size or shape of the breasts.
- Discharge from the nipple (other than milk!).
- Puckering or dimpling of the skin of the breast.
- Unusual pain or discomfort in or around the breast.

You are looking for *changes*, so learn how your breasts feel now.

Both boys and girls can be born with more than two nipples, either above or below the chest. Only the two nipples at armpit level on a girl will grow. The rest remain like children's nipples. Extra nipples should be left alone if milk comes from them during breastfeeding. Squeezing may cause infection. After a few days the milk will stop.

18

Dear Auntie,

One of my breasts is bigger than the other one. Am I normal? I am 17.

Gladys

Dear Gladys,

Yes, you are normal. Sometimes one breast grows faster than the other. They may catch up with each other, but many women always have one breast bigger than the other. Accepting our bodies is part of growing up. Sadly, some people are never happy with their bodies or faces. The beauty of humans is that we are all different. Imagine how boring life would be if we all looked the same!

If it really worries you, then wear a bra to fit the larger breast and pad the other side with soft cloth.

Female sex parts

A woman's sexual parts are not easy to see. Most of them are inside the body. Understanding how your body works is easier if you can at least see it. Many girls have never looked at their **genitals.** They think it is rude to look. Everyone should be proud, not ashamed, of their bodies. No girl or woman can see her own genitals properly unless she has a very long neck! So find a mirror and a quiet place where no-one will disturb you and look at your genitals. Identify the main features using the picture on page 20. Like faces, every **vulva** is different, but with the same features.

A girl's pubic and underarm hair begins to grow at about the same time as her breasts. Pubic hair grows in a triangle where a woman's legs meet and partly covers the vulva between the legs as far as the **anus.**

Folds of fleshy skin protect the **clitoris, urethra** and **vagina.** The skin on the inside is smooth, hairless and moist — like the inside of the mouth.

The clitoris is difficult to see. It feels like a small bean inside the inner lips of the vulva. The clitoris is the most sensitive part of a woman's body. Like the penis, the clitoris grows in size when a woman is sexually excited.

In front of the vagina is the urethra. The urethra is a tube 1 mm wide and difficult to see or feel. The narrow tube stays tight shut except when **urine** is flowing out. This prevents germs entering the **bladder** where urine is stored.

19

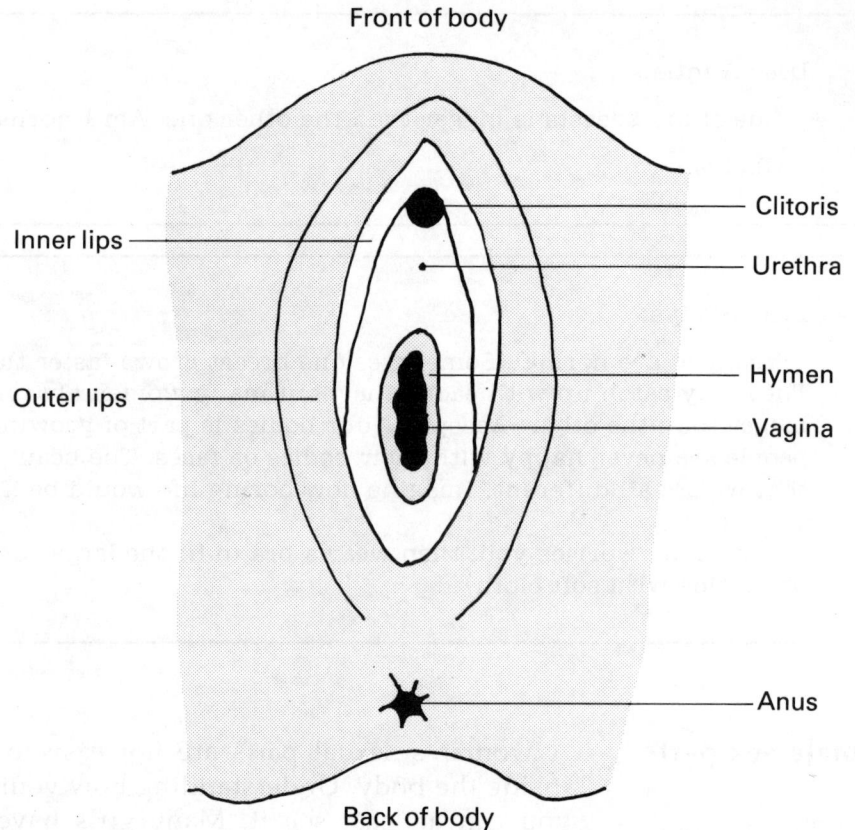

Front of body

Clitoris

Urethra

Inner lips

Outer lips

Hymen

Vagina

Anus

Back of body

Female genitals.

The vagina is a pink tube about 7 cm deep and 3 or 4 cm wide. It is soft, stretchy and moist. This is so that a penis can slip in during sex, and a baby can slip out at birth. The elastic skin stretches both ways during lovemaking to accept the erect penis. If a woman is forced to have sex her vagina will not be ready and it will be painful for her. During pregnancy the vagina becomes even more elastic ready for the birth of the baby.

The vagina has four purposes, all of them connected.
1   A tube for menstrual blood to flow through from the uterus.
2   A female part for sexual intercourse.
3   A tube to carry sperm to the ovum.
4   A tube for the birth of the baby.

The entrance to the vagina may be partly covered by thin skin called the **hymen**. Many people believe that the hymen shows if a girl is a virgin. Hymens vary as much as any part of the body. Some girls have a hymen that covers the whole vaginal opening with a very small hole for the menstrual blood to flow through. Other girls have very thin hymens. As a girl grows up the hymen stretches. If she takes part in active sports the hymen may stretch open, even though she is still a virgin.

In a very few women the hymen may completely cover the entrance to the vagina, and so prevent the menstrual flow from leaving the body. The young woman should visit a doctor who can open the hymen.

At the top of the vagina is the **cervix**. The cervix is a ring of muscle which holds the foetus in the **uterus** or **womb** during pregnancy. The hole through the cervix is the width of a needle. At birth the cervix opens and the baby slides through.

The uterus is a bag of muscle inside the abdomen about the size of an orange. It can only be felt during pregnancy when the uterus grows to hold a baby. The uterus protects the baby and then helps to push it out at birth.

The uterus has three openings. The lower opening goes into the vagina through the cervix. The openings on each side lead to two tubes about 1/2 cm wide and 5 cm long called the **fallopian tubes**. The fallopian tubes connect the uterus and the two ovaries. Each white **ovary** is about the size of a grape or a palm nut. The ovaries have two purposes. Ovaries store ova and they produce female sex hormones.

When a girl is born each of her ovaries contains between 200000 and 400000 ova — far more than any woman will ever need! Every 21 to 35 days after puberty one ovum is released. The two ovaries take it in turns to do this. This is called **ovulation**. One ovum is the size of a full stop. The end of the fallopian tube sucks the ovum inside it.

The ovum is pushed towards the uterus by tiny hairs inside the fallopian tube.

Fertilization happens in the fallopian tube. At ovulation the uterus is prepared for a possible fertilized ovum. The soft lining of the uterus fills with blood to make a nutritious bed about 1/2 cm thick for the embryo to grow in.

Periods

If fertilization does not occur then the lining of the uterus breaks up. The dead ovum, the cells from the lining of the uterus, mucus and about 3 spoonfuls of blood trickle out of the vagina as a **menstrual period** also called **menstruation** or a **period**.

When the lining of the uterus comes away during a period, some of the tiny blood vessels in the uterus bleed. This bleeding continues for three to eight days. The inside of the uterus heals quickly, ready to prepare a new lining.

Menstrual blood is not 'dirty' or 'unclean'. It is the same blood as when the finger is cut. When it comes out it is bright red. Like all blood, it turns brown in the air.

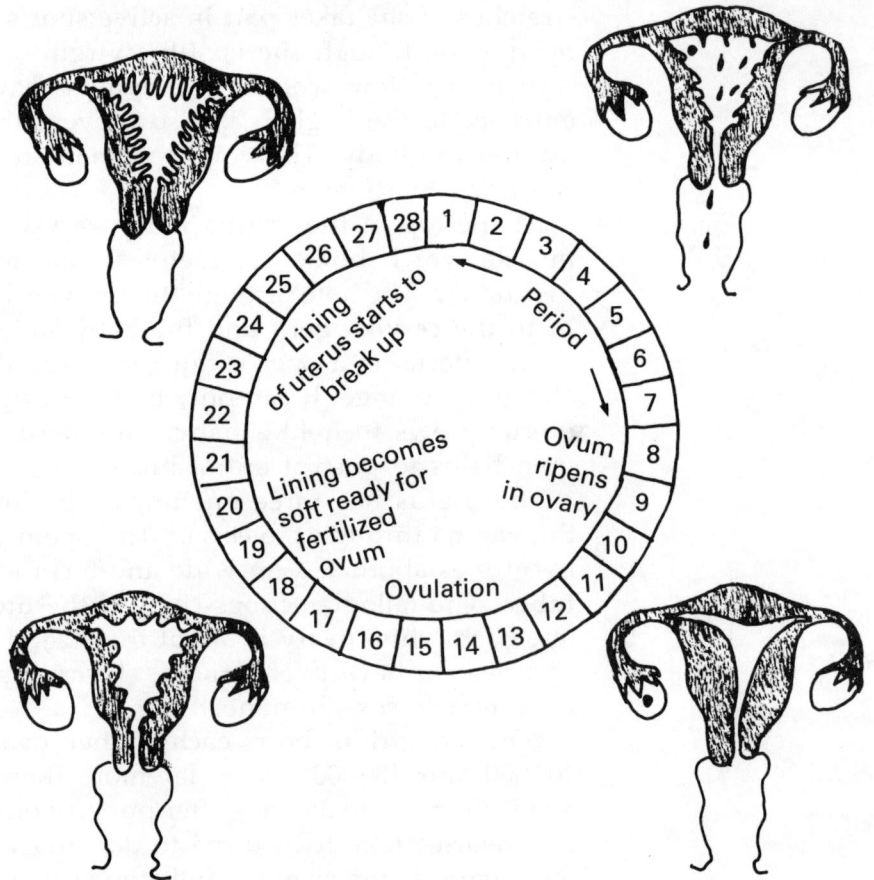

The uterus and menstruation.

A woman cannot control the flow of menstrual blood, as she can control urine. Nor does it pour out like urine.

Menstrual blood may appear to be more than 3 tablespoonfuls. This is because it is mixed up with mucus and cells from the uterus lining and it trickles out slowly. Some women bleed for only two days. Other women bleed for eight days. Most women notice that for the first day or two the bleeding is heavier and at the end of the period it is lighter. Very heavy periods are unhealthy, as too much blood loss can cause **anaemia**, or weak blood. Heavy bleeding may be a sign of an infection. Bleeding is 'heavy' if sanitary towels are soaked within an hour. No girl starts having periods with heavy bleeding, so she will soon learn what is a normal flow.

Women usually notice the start of a period when they go to the toilet. Some women notice a wet feeling in their pants when their periods begin. They do not feel the blood coming out.

Periods begin one or two years after the breasts have begun to grow. First periods may not happen every four weeks. Some young women have two or three months between each of their first few periods. A woman may be 20 years old before she has regular periods. Many women never have regular periods. Other women know that their periods always come exactly every 28, 30 or 35 days.

Ovulation happens 14 days before a period, whether a woman has a period every 26 or 36 days. Irregular periods do not make conception or pregnancy more difficult.

A woman has about 400 periods in her life and less if she has several pregnancies. Most of the thousands of ova in her ovaries are not needed.

For centuries people did not understand menstruation. They thought that it was a 'curse' on all woman. In some places women had to stay indoors, or could not touch food. Men could not go near menstruating women.

Even now, most women are embarrassed if anyone knows they are menstruating. Menstruation is not an illness. It is a normal part of every woman's life. Girls and women can continue doing all the things they do at any other time. They can take part in active sports, cook food, run, or go visiting.

Coping with periods, see Chapter 7, page 144.

Danger signs

Go to your clinic if you notice any of these.
- Bleeding between periods.

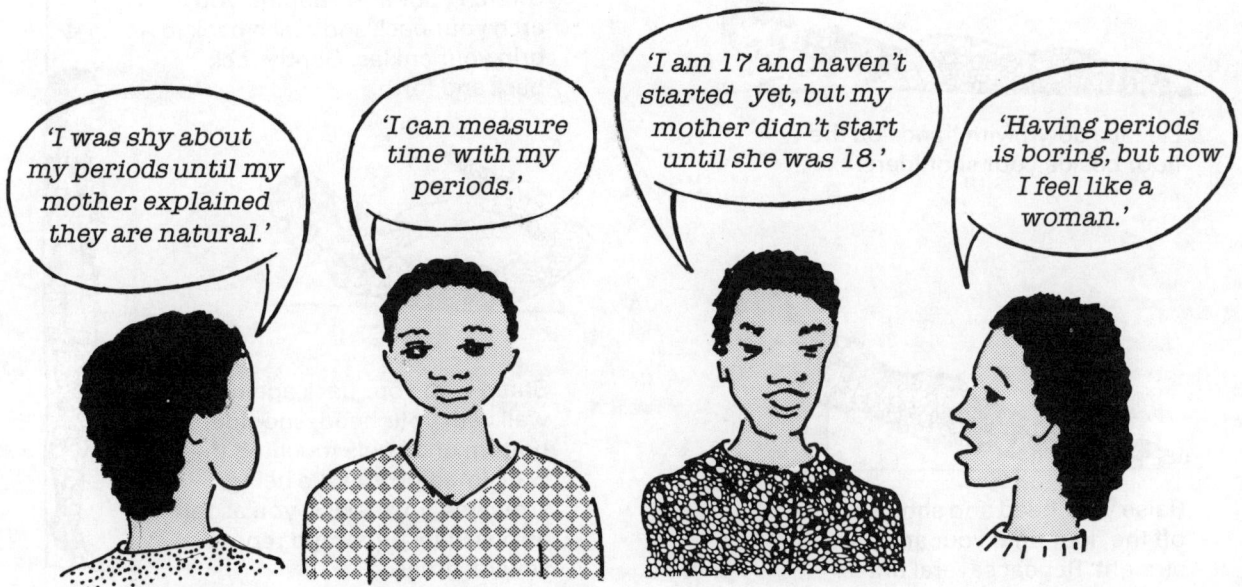

'I was shy about my periods until my mother explained they are natural.'

'I can measure time with my periods.'

'I am 17 and haven't started yet, but my mother didn't start until she was 18.'

'Having periods is boring, but now I feel like a woman.'

When do periods start?

- Bleeding after sexual intercourse.
- Heavy bleeding.
- Heavy bleeding with tiredness.
- Strong pains in the belly.

Moods and feelings

At different times during a woman's cycle the hormones produced by the ovaries may affect her moods and feelings. Some women feel especially happy at the time of ovulation. Other women feel depressed or tired just before or during a period. For a few days before a period the breasts and abdomen may feel full and heavy. This is because the fluid increases in these parts of the body. The feeling should go away when menstruation starts. Exercise will make the blood flow round the body quicker and so reduce the feeling.

Sometimes the contractions of the uterus during a period cause pain or discomfort. This can be helped by doing exercises. If the pain is bad then take two aspirin or paracetamol tablets and lie down with a bottle filled with hot water on the abdomen. If periods are always painful, then visit the clinic.

Some women also suffer from headaches, spots, tiredness or bad temper just before a period. When they remember that within a day or two it will improve, they usually feel better!

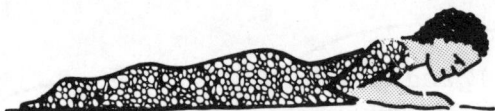

Lie face down with hands on the floor beside your shoulders.

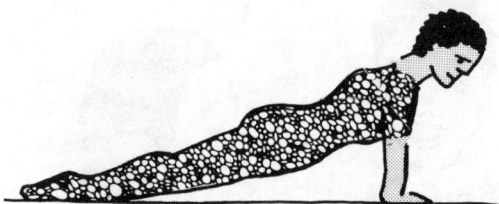

Lie flat face down on the floor. Stretch your arms behind you, arch your back and reach back to grip your ankles. Gently rock back and forth.

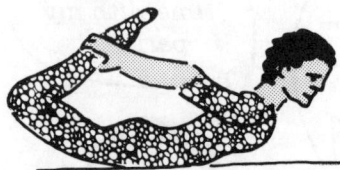

Raise your head and shoulders off the floor until your arms are straight. Repeat several times.

Stand with your back against a wall with your head, shoulders, bottom and heels touching the wall. Imagine you are being stretched up, making you as tall as possible. Relax and repeat several times.

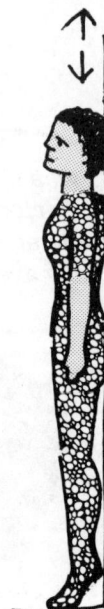

Exercises for period pains.

24

Dear Auntie,

I have just started my menstrual periods. What foods can I eat during a period? Can other people tell when I have a period?

Fatima

Dear Fatima,

You can eat any of the foods you enjoy at any other time of the month. Your body works in the same way whether you are menstruating or not. Eggs, meat, fresh vegetables, nuts — none of these will harm you. Green leaf vegetables, peanuts, oranges and ripe bananas are especially good for women — they help to strengthen the blood.

No-one knows if you are having a period unless you tell them. All normal women menstruate, so try not to be embarrassed about it.

Menopause

From about 40 years a woman's ovaries produce less sex hormones. She stops menstruating and can no longer become pregnant. Sex hormones affect the whole body so she may notice other changes, too. Her hair will grow white and her skin has more wrinkles.

A few women become depressed, or they cry for no reason. Other women feel tired, or have headaches or their bones and muscles ache.

Some women have 'hot flushes' when the head and upper body feel like a fever for a few minutes. Afterwards the woman feels cold and damp.

The vagina and vulva may become dry which can cause soreness or infection. During sexual intercourse she can use a special cream or jelly.

The **menopause** can be helped if the women eats well and keeps fit. Foods like green leaves, milk, eggs and butter are good for bones. Talking to other women of the same age or older helps.

Menopause does not have to be a difficult time for women. Younger women may be frightened, but it is a natural part of being a woman. Most women have no unpleasant symptoms. They feel relieved that they no longer have to worry about unwanted pregnancy. They can enjoy making love without using contraception.

No woman can assume that she is infertile until she has had no periods for two years. Until that time she should continue to use contraceptives to prevent pregnancy. Some women have periods

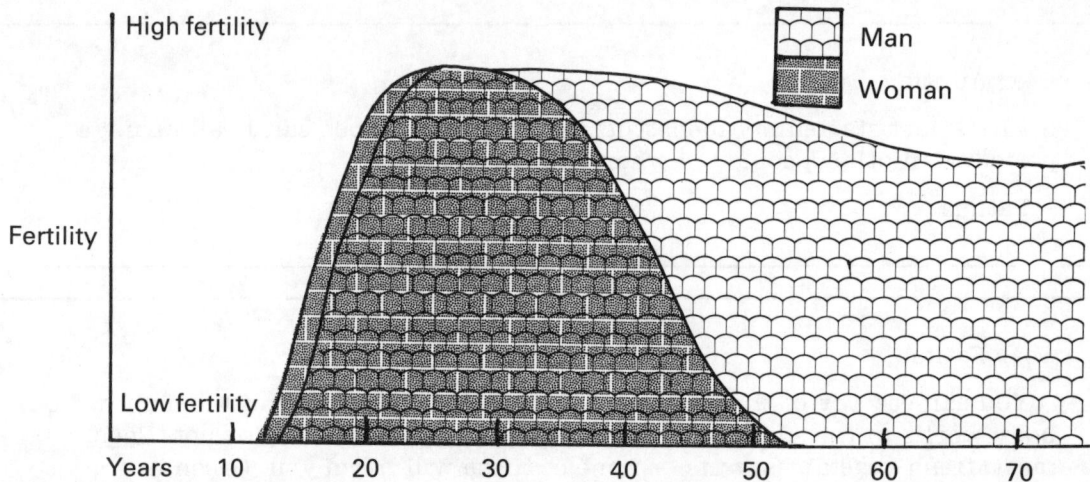

High fertility

Fertility

Low fertility

Years   10   20   30   40   50   60   70

Man
Woman

Age graph of fertility.

again after they have not menstruated for a whole year.

The menopause can begin at 35 years or at 55 years. It can last from two years to six years. Every woman is different. The age of puberty has no effect on the age of menopause.

Puberty and boys

Puberty in boys is on average a year later than in girls. Even though the sexual parts are easy to see, many men do not understand how their bodies work.

At puberty a boy grows very fast in height. His feet may appear too big for his body but he quickly catches up with them. His chest and shoulders grow wider and his muscles grow harder and stronger.

Voice

The '**Adam's apple**' enlarges and can be seen sticking out of the neck below the chin. The voice 'breaks' and sounds deeper. This may happen in a few days, or take several months. The voice is at first difficult to control: it may squeak one minute and sound very low the next. Women have small Adam's apples, and their voices deepen a little at puberty.

Skin

The skin all over the body goes through changes. Extra sweat is made in the armpits, feet and around the genitals. After physical games like football young people smell unpleasant if they do not wash. The body also sweats when just sitting still. Over active oil glands in the skin may cause **acne** (See Chapter 7, page 141.)

Hair	Hair gradually starts to grow in the armpits, around the genitals and on the face. At first the new hair is soft, but it gradually grows stronger and thicker. Some men also have hairy chests and legs.
Nipples	During puberty the sex hormones are so busy in the body that they may work too hard. Boys sometimes get tender or swollen nipples. After a few months the hormones settle down and the 'breasts' disappear. Boys should not worry that they are becoming women!
Male sex parts	Even baby boys discover that the penis feels good to touch. If stroked gently even a baby's penis grows hard. And when hit hard it hurts a lot!

At puberty the penis grows larger. Like all parts of the body penises vary in size and shape. They are all different like eyes and ears, though they all work in the same way.

The penis is smooth, hairless and dry, and made of spongy tissue full of blood vessels. Most of the time the penis is soft and the blood flows in and out. When a man is close to a woman he is attracted to, or thinks about her, the blood flow into the penis increases. The blood fills the spongy tissue and the penis grows longer, hard and stands up. The penis has to be erect for sexual intercourse. After **ejaculation** the muscles relax. The blood flows out and the penis goes soft again.

Most penises are about 5 to 8 cm long when soft and grow to about 15 cm when erect. Penises that are small when they are soft grow more than penises that are normally larger. So they all end

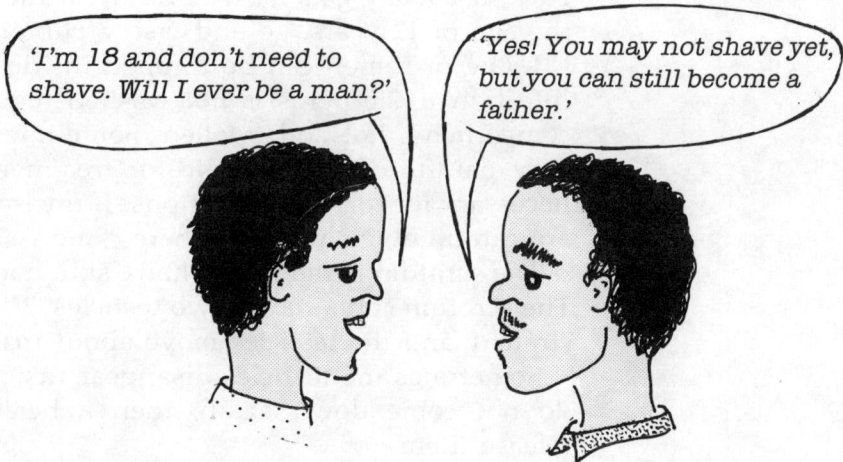

'I'm 18 and don't need to shave. Will I ever be a man?'

'Yes! You may not shave yet, but you can still become a father.'

When do boys start to shave?

27

up about the same size at erection. The angle of the **erection** varies from one penis to the next. Some penises stand up more than others. The size of the penis has no effect on sexual pleasure for the man or woman, or the ability to father children.

Temperature also affects the size of the penis. In cold weather the penis and the testicles contract to be close to the body. In warm weather they relax and hang down lower.

There are no medicines or tools for increasing the size of a penis. Anyone advertising such things is lying, and just wants your money.

The head of the penis, or **glans**, is the most sensitive part of a man's body. A white cream called **smegma** is produced on the glans. This protects the glans and helps the **foreskin** to slide smoothly over it. The smell of smegma excites some women during lovemaking, just as the smell of women excites men.

At the tip of the penis is the small opening to the urethra that runs up the inside of the penis. Inside the abdomen the urethra branches into two smaller tubes. One tube leads to the bladder and carries urine. The other tube leads to the **testicles** and carries **semen** and **sperm**.

All boys are born with a fold of skin around the end of the penis. This is the foreskin, which protects the sensitive glans. During washing, or lovemaking, the foreskin can be pulled back revealing the glans. Up until about two years from birth the foreskin is still attached to the glans. The penis can be damaged if the foreskin is forced back.

Some men and boys have been circumcised − their foreskins have been cut off. (See page 30.) Circumcision makes no difference to a man's sexual powers. When a penis is erect a circumcised penis and an uncircumcised penis look almost the same.

The foreskin can sometimes be too tight and painful to pull back. It usually gets looser in time. If the foreskin is still tight at the age of 12 years, go and visit a clinic.

Urine or semen can be trapped inside the foreskin and cause infection if the penis is not washed regularly. The foreskin becomes itchy, hot and swollen. Sometimes there is pus and it is very painful. Go to a clinic for treatment. Circumcision is not necessary for foreskin infections. If uncircumcised men and boys are careful about washing there is no risk of infection.

The **scrotum** is the bag of hairy skin hanging behind the penis. The scrotum contains the two testicles. The skin of the scrotum is stretchy and the testicles move about inside.

Sometimes the testicles disappear inside the abdomen. If they do not come down again, then a health worker can usually release them.

The scrotum also controls the temperature of the testicles. Sperm can only be produced in temperatures cooler than the rest of the body. In cold weather the scrotum contracts, bringing the testicles nearer the body to warm them. The scrotum also contracts when the man is sexually excited or nervous.

In warm weather the scrotum is relaxed, so that the testicles hang down and keep cool. Some men are infertile because they wear tight jeans which make their testicles too warm!

One side of the scrotum is often lower than the other. This is normal.

The two testicles are inside the scrotum. They are the size of palm nuts, or small plums, though their size varies. Small or large testicles work equally well. Testicles grow larger about a year before the penis does.

Testicles produce **sex hormones**. At about 12 years the hormones stimulate the body to begin puberty.

Testicles also produce sperm. Sperm can only be seen with a **microscope**. Sperm take about two months to grow, but many millions are made every day. Testicles make new sperm until a man dies. Even a man of 95 years can make a woman pregnant!

The sperm wait in long coiled tubes called the **epididymis**, which are wrapped around the testicles. Each epididymis is as thick as human hair and 6 m long! If the man does not ejaculate for several weeks, the sperm are absorbed back into his body and fresh sperm are made.

Testicles are very sensitive and boys soon learn to protect them from injury. Some young men feel pressure in their testicles if they are sexually excited for a long time. This does no harm to the testicles and the feeling soon goes away.

Go to a clinic if there is any unusual lump, pain or swelling in the testicles. This may be a **rupture**, or a **cyst**. Very rarely it is cancer, which can be cured with early treatment.

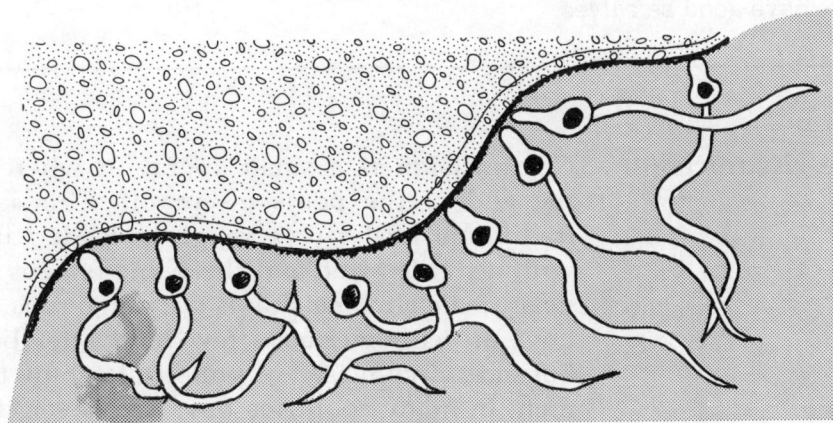

Sperm growing in the epididymis.

Each testicle has a **sperm duct**, or **vas**, leading from the epididymis up into the body. The vas are about 40 cm long and 2-3 mm thick. When a man is sexually excited several million sperm are pushed up the vas to the **prostate gland**. This is a bag the size of a palm nut where semen is made. Semen is the sticky white fluid that comes out of the penis when a man ejaculates. Semen helps the sperm to move. At the climax of sexual intercourse the muscles around the penis contract and the semen squirts out. There is about a small spoonful.

Dear Auntie,

I am 17 years old and I have only one testicle. I am worried this is going to affect my sex life. Will I be able to make children?

Harry

Dear Harry,

You probably do have two testicles, but one of them is still inside your abdomen. Until puberty the testes can move up and down freely between the scrotum and the inside of the body. But sometimes, one or both testes remain inside. Doctors can perform a small operation to bring the testicle down into the scrotum.

Testes inside the body will still produce male sex hormones so that a boy turns into a man at puberty. But sperm can only be produced at a temperature lower than 37°C. This is why the scrotum hangs outside the body where it is cooler.

One testicle can make enough sperm to fertilize an ovum. Many men have lost one testicle through accident or disease. They still become fathers, and have good sex lives.

Male circumcision Circumcision is a small operation where the foreskin covering the end of the penis is cut off. This is done by a doctor, a traditional healer or a religious leader. If a boy is circumcised with a sterile knife and the penis is kept clean while the wound heals, male circumcision is not dangerous. In some societies baby boys are circumcised a few days after birth. In other societies boys are circumcised at puberty to show that they are now adult men. In many countries boys are never circumcised.

The penis works equally well whether a man is circumcised or not. After circumcision the skin of the glans becomes slightly

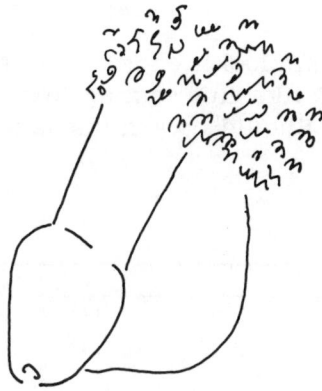

Circumcised penis.   *Uncircumcised penis.*

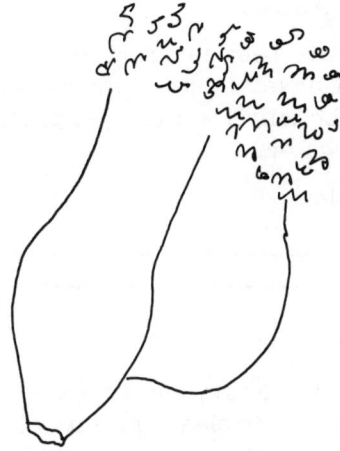

thicker and tougher. Uncircumcised men and boys are not 'unclean,' though they must wash inside their foreskins, as germs can be trapped there.

Female circumcision

In some countries women are circumcised, which means the clitoris is cut off. A woman can still have children, but she will not enjoy making love so much. In other countries the clitoris and the lips of the vulva are cut off, so that the woman has no wet, smooth skin left. The sides of the vulva are sewn together, leaving only a small hole through which urine and the menstrual flow pass.

Depending on the local custom, circumcision is performed at any age between birth and puberty.

Female circumcision is often performed by the local midwife who has neither medicines to relieve pain nor knowledge of germ free conditions. During the operation the urethra may be damaged. Sexual intercourse will be painful because the sewn up vagina is too small for a man's penis. The scarred skin tears or has to be cut. Later when she gives birth to her baby, more cutting is needed because the hole is too small and will not stretch. Female circumcision often leads to dangerous infection, bleeding and blood poisoning. This may either kill the woman, or make her unable to conceive babies.

Female circumcision is a very old but harmful custom. In many countries the practice is now illegal, but the custom will not stop until men and women understand the dangers.

31

Dear Auntie,

I have been married for a year. I am looking forward to getting pregnant, but I have noticed some white stuff, like glue coming from my vagina. Could this be why I am not yet pregnant? Should I wash inside my vagina with soap and water?

Helen

Dear Helen,

During ovulation, half way between two periods, there is more vaginal mucus. It is clear and stretches like the white of a hen's egg. This makes lovemaking comfortable and helps the sperm to swim up through the uterus towards the ovum. During the rest of the month the vagina secretes mucus which is tacky, not stretchy.

Keep a calendar marking the days when you have a period and the days when you have this slippery mucus. After a few months you will be able to work out the days when you ovulate (see Chapter 5, page 97.) If you want to get pregnant then these three or four days are the best time to have sex.

If the discharge smells unpleasant, or the vulva is inflamed and itchy, then there may be an infection. Go and visit your clinic. But all women have natural mucus from their vaginas and vulvas.

Washing inside the vagina with soap and water is not a good idea as it can cause infections, by destroying the natural mucus. This mucus helps prevent infections. Some women find that even washing their vulvas with soap makes them dry and itchy. The 'white stuff' you notice is quite natural.

Activities

1 Copy the diagram of either male or female sex organs. Without looking at the book, label the parts.

2 Draw a picture of how you see yourself. Draw a picture of how you would like to be. Draw a picture of your best friend. (You do not have to be good at drawing!) Compare your pictures with your friend's pictures. Discuss the differences between how you see yourself and how others see you. Does this help you to feel more positive about yourself?

3 Divide the group into four separate groups. Each group write a list of either the advantages or disadvantages of being a man or a woman. After 20 minutes the groups should compare their lists. What things would you like to change about male and female roles in society? Are some people's lives restricted by their roles?

4 Make a role play about men and women who model themselves on film star or magazine advertisements, and other people who act naturally.

CHAPTER 3
Sexual intercourse

Boys and girls change into men and women so that they can reproduce more boys and girls, who will grow into men and women.

A woman needs the help of a man to make a baby. One ovum is ready to be fertilized in the woman every menstrual cycle. This ovum can only grow into a baby if it is fertilized by a man's sperm. The sperm have to reach the ovum in the fallopian tubes. This is where the penis is so useful. The man puts his sperm into the woman's vagina with his penis. This is called **sexual intercourse**, the **sex act, making love, coitus** or **sex**. Animals do this too, but only when the female can get pregnant. Men and women are different because they can make love at any time because they enjoy it, even if they do not want a baby.

Sexual intercourse is the nearest two people in love can get to being one person. If a couple love each other, then sex is 'making love'. Making love seals and encourages their love for each other both in mind and body. Once a couple are sealed together by marriage and sex, they continue to have sex in order to maintain their love.

In books and films sex is always wonderful and everyone knows how to do it perfectly from the beginning. But no-one knows how to ride a bicycle or drive a car without some practice. Although people have been having sex since time began, many couples know nothing about it before they try. Learning about the theory of sex helps people to enjoy it later.

If making love is to be a pleasure then it requires a loving relationship and desire from *both* the man and the woman. No man or woman should ever make love just because their partner wants to.

Making love needs plenty of time and patience. It cannot be rushed or hurried. Sex can take only five minutes, but the more time a couple has, the more pleasure they can give and receive.

Comfort, and no risk of being disturbed are important. The back of a car is too small, and no-one can relax comfortably on bare ground with stones digging into them!

Some couples enjoy music while they are making love. Others

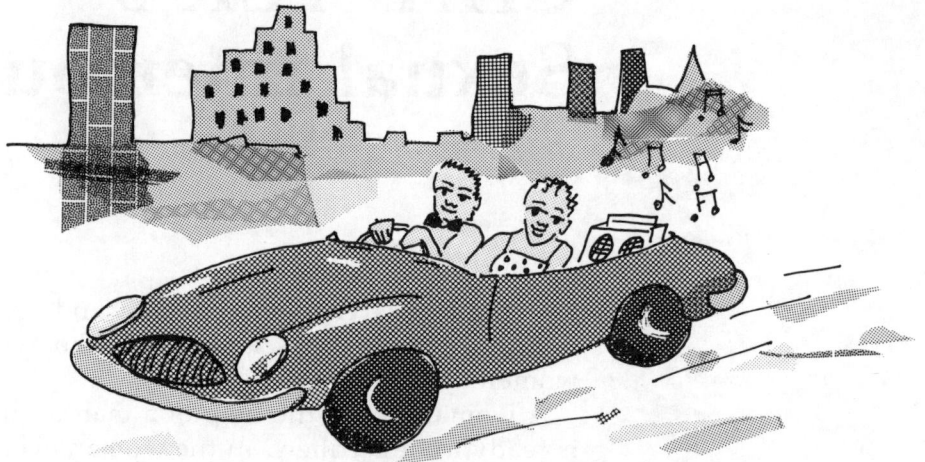

Is real life like this?

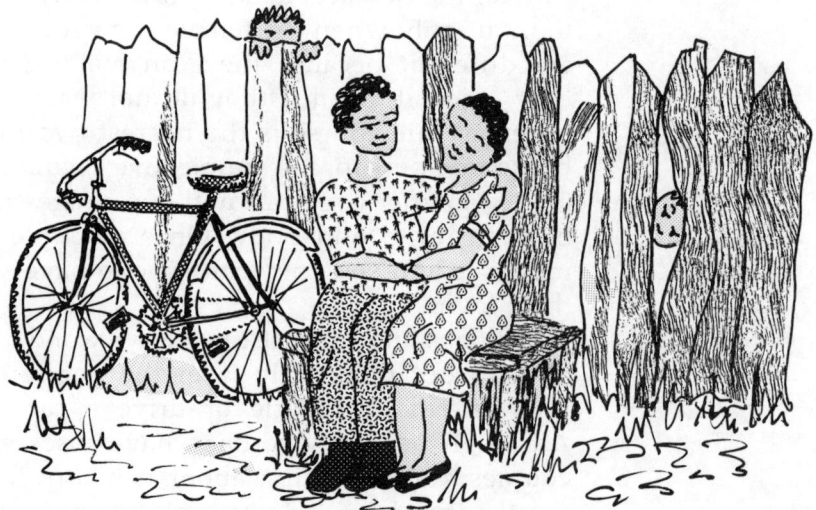

Or more like this?

prefer to listen to each other talking, whispering, laughing or even singing.

Strictly speaking, sexual intercourse begins when the penis enters the vagina. But **foreplay** before intercourse is part of making love.

Stroking, kissing and fondling each other creates a desire for sexual intercourse. This is why parents worry about their teenage children 'going too far'. Once a couple start making love, it is

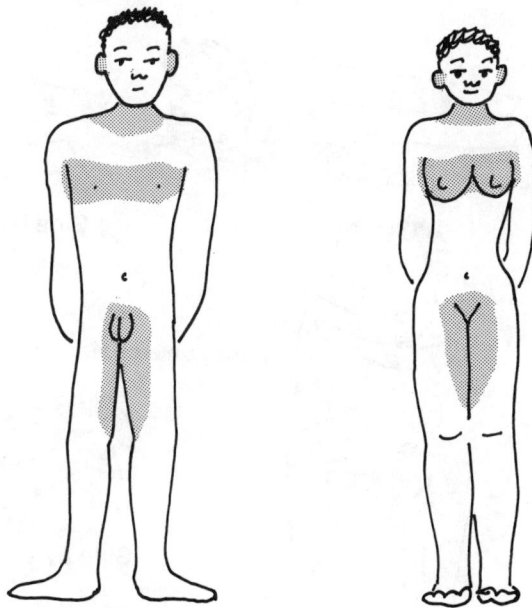

Erogenous areas.

very difficult for them to stop before intercourse.

Anything is acceptable if both partners enjoy it. Kissing, licking, gentle biting, sucking, stroking and squeezing. All the senses are increased when a couple are sexually excited. The whole body becomes more sensitive to touch. Some parts of the body, such as the genitals, lips and nipples are extra sensitive. These are called erogenous areas.

The most sensitive part of a man is the glans, and the most sensitive part of a woman is the clitoris. Men and women enjoy having these parts stroked and caressed.

Both the man and the woman give off special smells during lovemaking which further excite each other. The breathing and heart beat increase and their nipples grow erect. The man's penis grows erect (see Chapter 2, page 29).

The changes in a woman are not so visible. Blood rushes to her genitals in the same way that it does with a man. The vulva becomes larger and the vagina expands. Her clitoris grows hard like an erect penis. The vagina is ready to accept the penis when it is lubricated by slippery colourless mucus. If the penis is put in too soon, then the vagina may not be wet and relaxed inside, and the woman will feel pain.

The woman can lie on her back with her legs apart and the man on top with his weight resting on his elbows, or the woman can be on top, or the couple may lie side by side. Some couples

Man on top

Side by side facing

Sitting on a chair

Side by side, man behind woman

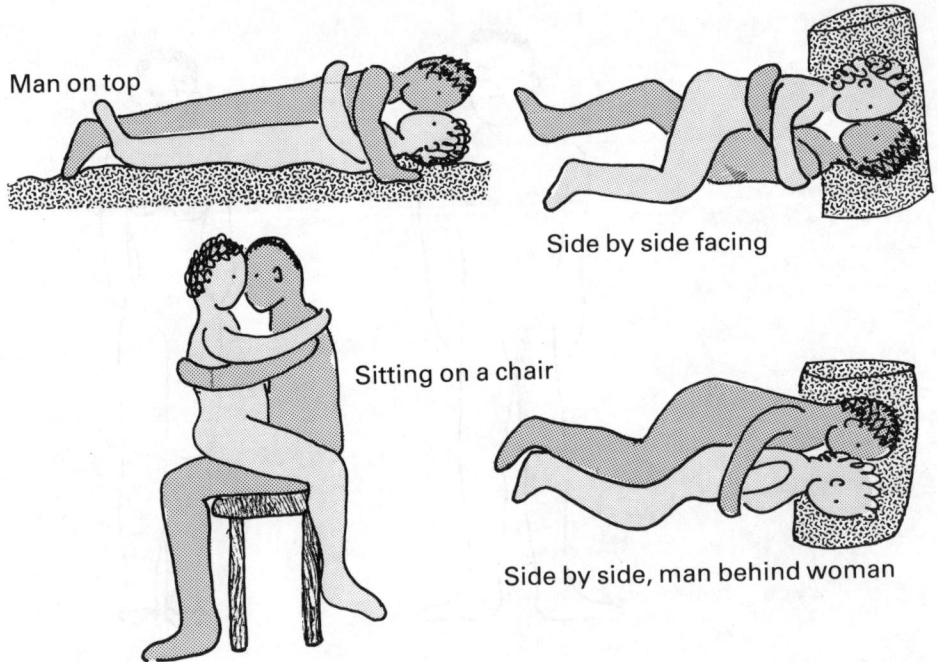

Different positions for making love.

prefer making love sitting on a chair, lying on the floor, or standing up. The man can enter from behind and stimulate the woman's clitoris with his hands.

There are many different positions and couples can vary their position. They can experiment to find out which they enjoy most.

The man pushes the penis slowly into the vagina with small thrusts, opening up the vagina gently. The woman may like to guide it in with her hand.

Once the penis is inside the vagina one or both partners move their hips so that the penis slides in and out in a rhythmical movement. This can be fast or slow, depending on the mood of the couple. This is coitus, or being together.

The vagina does not always produce enough natural mucus even when the woman is excited. This can be uncomfortable for both the man and the woman. Cream, oil, spit or jelly all work well. Do not use petroleum jelly with a condom or a cap as it rots the rubber. Some condoms are already lubricated.

Orgasm is the climax of sexual excitement for both the man and the woman and occurs after a few minutes, depending on how excited the couple are.

The couple feel a wave of intense muscular spasms in their genitals. A tingling warm feeling may spread through the body right to the toes and fingers. They feel intense pleasure followed by happy relaxation.

Every orgasm for every person is different. Sometimes an orgasm lasts a couple of seconds. At other times lovemaking lasts an hour and the orgasm is longer and more intense.

After making love the couple feel warm and close. They may want to make love again. A woman can have several orgasms in a row, but a man has to wait a while between orgasms. The number of orgasms in one day or night is not always a measure of a couple's relationship. One good loving orgasm is better then three orgasms without any love or communication between the couple.

One partner may reach orgasm before the other, or they may have an orgasm at the same time. If the man ejaculates first, then he can stimulate the woman's clitoris with his fingers. They should not worry if either of them does not reach orgasm. Being close and understanding is more important.

Fear and anxiety cause more problems in sex than true physical problems. If either partner worries about lovemaking then it may be tense and not so enjoyable! Both partners must feel relaxed and understand what is happening.

If sexual intercourse is to be a pleasure for both partners there must be a loving relationship and desire in both the man and woman.

Building a good sexual relationship takes time, which is why having sex with strangers is never satisfactory. Like walking or

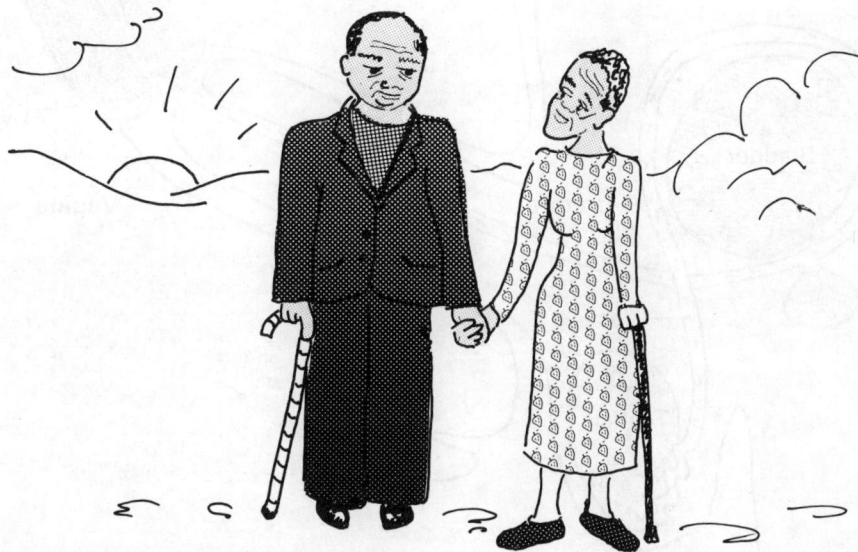

'Building a relationship takes time.'

talking, patience and practice are needed. Both partners must be aware of each others needs and be aware that sex can always be improved. The more good feelings you can give to another person, the more will be returned. Making love may not be very exciting the first time, but it should get better and better.

Ejaculation

When a man has an erection the sperm move up from the testicles along the vas to the prostate gland near the bladder. This gland produces the semen which gives the sperm energy to swim. The urethra leading to the bladder closes so that urine and semen cannot mix.

At ejaculation the muscles around the penis force the semen out in a quick squirt. Each ejaculation of semen is about a teaspoon (5 ml) of sticky white fluid containing 200 million to 400 million sperm. Sperm are so small they can only be seen with a strong microscope. If a man has several ejaculations in one night

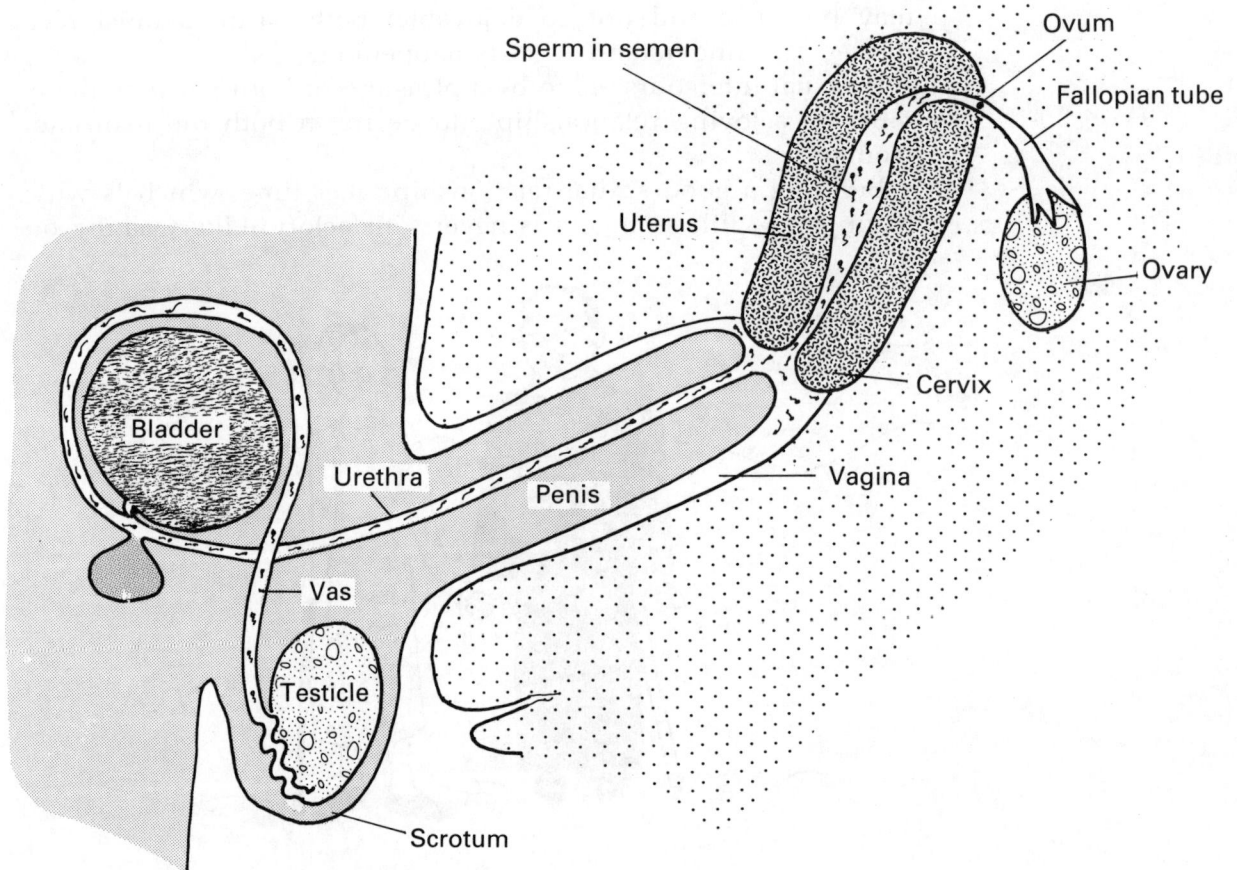

The sperms' journey from testicle to uterus.

the sperm will be reduced. But the man can still make a woman pregnant — only one sperm is needed to make a baby! The testicles manufacture 1000 to 2000 sperm per second, day and night.

When a man ejaculates, the woman cannot feel the semen inside her. Most of the semen flows back out of the vagina but many millions of sperm will already be on their way towards the ovum. The sperm swim in the woman's mucus. At ovulation the vagina and uterus produce extra mucus which the sperm swim through easily. The sperm swim up the uterus to find an ovum. Sperm swim about 3 cm an hour and can live for up to seven days. Most sperm die and come out of the vagina.

The penis goes soft and limp immediately after ejaculating. If the man is young, he can have another erection in a few minutes. As men get older it takes longer.

Dear Auntie,

I am 18 years old and I worry day and night because I have a very small penis. I am so ashamed of it that I avoid urinating in public toilets. I have never had sexual intercourse because I am afraid of girls — they might laugh at my small penis.

John

Dear John,

This is a common worry among young men. The size of a penis bears no relation to its power, capabilities or the sensations felt by either the man or woman during sex. Women are not attracted to men by the size of their penises! It is the kindness and good humour of a man that wins their hearts. Girls are not thinking about your penis when they meet you. Just act naturally with them and think of them as people to talk to, not as women to sleep with. Sex can come later when you are a grown married man.

Women have many different sizes and shapes of breasts, so why should all men's penises be the same?

If you have erections then there is nothing physically wrong with you. But if you worry about your penis then you may lose your confidence and it could stop functioning.

Dear Auntie,

My ejaculation seems weak and I don't produce enough semen to satisfy my partners. I only produce about one spoon the first time and I usually dry up after two rounds. Are there any tablets I can take to increase my semen production?

Sizwe

Dear Sizwe,

No man produces more than a tablespoon of semen at each ejaculation. A teaspoon is quite normal and enough semen to carry up to 400 million sperms. The prostate gland takes a few hours to produce more semen so you cannot expect the same amount after a few minutes. A woman's sexual satisfaction depends on her partner's caring attitude and thoughtfulness towards her needs, not on the quantity of semen.

Many couples are embarrassed to speak to each other during lovemaking, but talking is the best way of finding out what your partner enjoys most. This is one reason why sex with many partners is never satisfactory. The longer a couple know each other, the better their lovemaking will become. But only if they keep communicating and guide each other in the right direction.

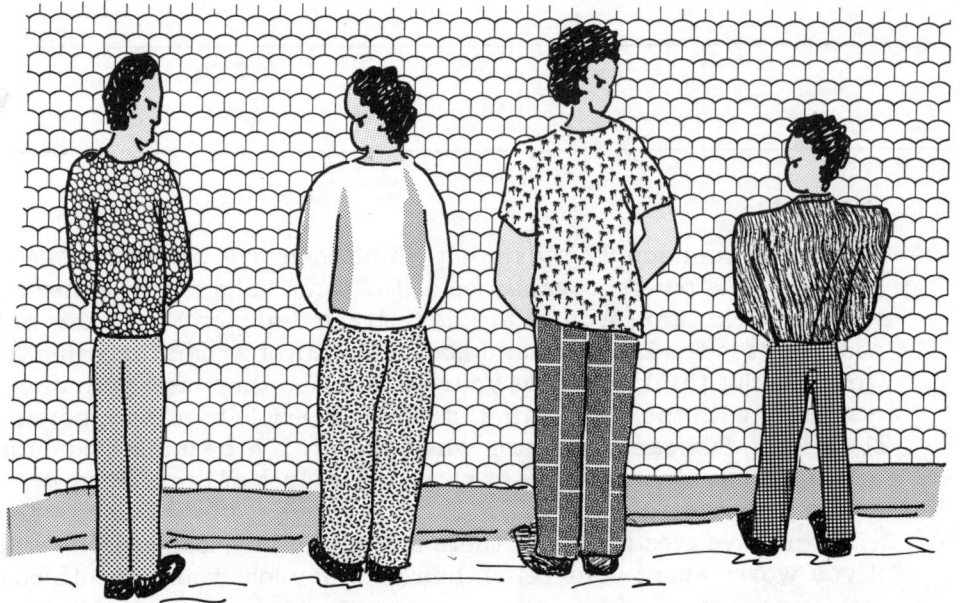

'Penis size is not important to a man's fertility or sexual power.'

Fertilization

After ejaculation millions of sperm find their way to the fallopian tube where an ovum may be waiting. Fertilization always occurs in a fallopian tube. The first sperm to reach the ovum joins with it and fertilization occurs. Every single sperm is different and every single ovum is different. They all contain characteristics of the man or the woman, but in different combinations. When the sperm and the ovum are joined the new baby will have some characteristics of each parent. Brothers and sisters are not identical because each ovum and sperm are different.

As soon as fertilization occurs the fertilized ovum travels along the fallopian tube to the uterus where it will grow into the soft lining prepared for it. Hormones are released to prepare the body for pregnancy. Ovulation and menstruation stop. Mucus blocks off the narrow passage through the cervix to keep out infections.

Every act of sexual intercourse can end in pregnancy. Once a sperm gets into the vagina there is nothing stopping it reaching an ovum. If the woman wants to have a baby, that is fine. But if she does not want to be pregnant, then she and her partner must think ahead and use contraception. If you want a baby, read the next chapter. If you do not, read Chapter 5 on child spacing and contraception.

Dear Auntie,

Is it true that if a couple make love during the first half of the menstrual cycle then the baby will be a boy, and if they make love during the second half then they will have a girl?

Ali

Dear Ali,

No, this is not true. Parents cannot choose to conceive a boy or a girl. The woman's ovum has no **gender** — it is neither male nor female. The man's sperm carry the gender of the future baby. Half the sperm are male and half are female and they are all mixed up. Every baby has an equal chance of being male or female. Neither parent has any control over the gender of their children. Fathers should not blame mothers for the gender of their children.

Dear Auntie,

I have missed three periods and sometimes I feel sick. I do not think I can be pregnant because although my boyfriend and I have been very close we have never had proper sexual intercourse. I know my hymen has not broken.

If I am pregnant, will my baby be able to get out? Are there any tablets I can take to break the hymen?

Annie

Dear Annie,

A woman can become pregnant without having full sexual intercourse. If a man ejaculates near the vagina then the sperm can still swim through the vaginal mucus up into the uterus.

Do not worry about the hymen. This rarely breaks, it actually stretches. During pregnancy the skin in and around the vagina becomes elastic so that your baby will be able to get out. There are no tablets or medicines to make it stretch further. Any medicines could be dangerous for the unborn baby.

Virginity

Everyone is born a **virgin**, both boys and girls. The only difference is that girls have hymens which may have to stretch for the penis to enter. Many girls have thin hymens that are stretched by active sports, or using tampons so that their first sexual experience is not painful. This does not mean that a girl has lied about being a virgin. Some women are so afraid of the pain of losing their virginity that the muscles around the vagina tighten. This makes it impossible to have intercourse. Relaxation is important. The most comfortable way to stretch a hymen ready for intercourse is gradually with the fingers. A woman can do this for herself, or her partner can do it as part of their lovemaking before they embark on intercourse. It may take a few days to stretch it gently. Even after this the penis may still be a tight fit at first. If the man does not force himself on the woman and is gentle and loving, then the woman will enjoy herself so much she may hardly notice.

If a man wants to know if the woman he is to marry is a virgin then he must trust what she tells him. There is no way of telling whether a man or woman is a virgin just by looking at them.

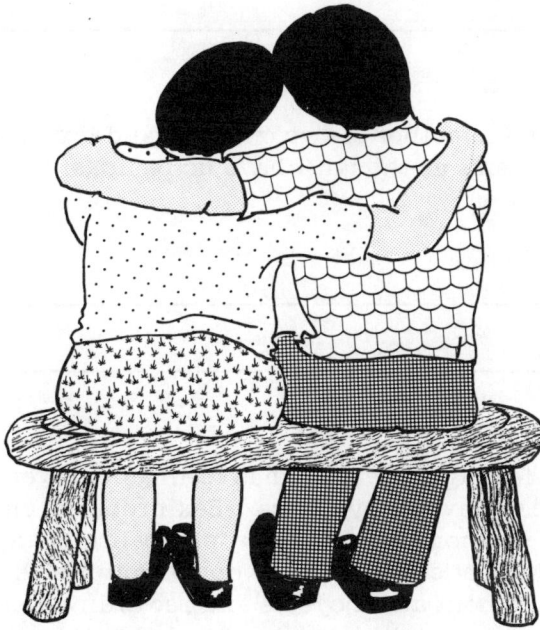

'Hugging is as important as sex.'

Dear Auntie,

I am 23 and about to be married. How often is it normal to make love? Are there times when my wife and I should not make love?

Tendai

Dear Tendai,

Whatever a couple feel is right for them, is normal. A young couple just married may make love once or twice a day. An older couple may make love once a week, or once a month. As people get older they may feel like sex less often as other things such as children or work take up time and energy.

Frequent sexual intercourse is not the most important part of a loving relationship. Just as important is plenty of hugging and cuddling to show your love for one another. If your wife does not want intercourse, do not turn your back and ignore her. Give her a friendly hug.

There is no time when you cannot make love. Some couples do not want to make love when the woman is menstruating, but there is no reason why you cannot make love then. Many couples do.

The only time when women should not make love is just after delivering a baby. The ante-natal clinic can advise when it is safe again.

Dear Auntie,

I am 23 years old and a mother of two children and my problem is I have never enjoyed sex. It seems as though I have no feelings. Is this my fault or my husband's?

Sally

Dear Sally,

Of course you have feelings! Everyone has feelings, but you have to find them. Every woman can have enjoyable sex. Sex problems among married couples are far more common than many people realise. Many people assume that they know the skills of sex when they don't. Couples should not go through married life without an enjoyable and rewarding sexual relationship.

First you have to be honest with your husband about your present lack of feelings. Try not to think of this problem as anyone's 'fault.' This is a negative approach and produces guilty feelings between you.

Do you and your husband talk openly about sex and what you enjoy? Perhaps he makes loves too quickly, and then rolls over and goes to sleep.

To start with, try not to have sexual intercourse for a couple of weeks. Spend some time each evening just holding and touching each other. Stroke each other's bodies all over. Talk to each other about what you feel, or guide each other's hands. Your husband will certainly become aroused, but no harm will come to him if he waits and learns how to please you. He will enjoy making love more too if he knows that you are also enjoying it. So ask him to be patient.

Only when you are really enjoying stroking each other and you absolutely have to go further, should you have sexual intercourse.

Wet dreams

Boys and men often have 'wet dreams' during the night. In the morning they wake and find a damp patch of semen on the bedclothes. They have ejaculated while asleep. They may remember having had a pleasant or sexy dream about women. Wet dreams are a natural and harmless part of a man's life, whether young or old. Semen can be washed out of the bedclothes with soap and cold water.

Many people believe that wet dreams are a way of releasing surplus sperm and semen. In fact too much semen is never made, and nor can a man use up too much. The body makes more sperm and semen as it is released. Wet dreams occur because adolescent men think about women a lot. Older men may have less wet dreams because their sexual thoughts are fulfilled by their wives.

Many men and boys wake in the mornings with erections, though they may not remember having a dream about sex.

During adolescence young men can be frequently embarrassed by having an erection at the wrong time! They may see or think about an attractive woman. Sometimes an erection happens when the genitals are accidentally touched. The best way of reducing an unwanted erection is to think very hard about something else. Not ejaculating after an erection does not harm the body.

Girls and women also have dreams about men and sex, but as they do not ejaculate they may not remember. They may wake up thinking 'That was a nice dream'. Dreams and thoughts about the opposite sex are quite natural and show that the brain is involved in sex as much as the body.

Sex is not just about genitals and sexual parts of the body. The mind and emotions are just as important. Falling in love involves liking someone's personality and character as well as being physically attracted.

Myth: 'If a man does not have regular sex he will suffer from backache. Eventually his testes will burst.'

Truth: Young men and old men do not suffer physically if they do not have sex with women. Any excess sperm or semen is re-absorbed into the body. Or a man can masturbate, or he may have wet dreams.

Myth: To find out if a man is sterile, put some semen into a jar of water. If the semen sinks then the man is fertile. If the semen floats then he is infertile.

Truth: The only way to know if there are sperm in semen is with a microscope. Infertility among men is not common. If a couple have been trying to conceive for two years without success then they should visit a clinic together.

Masturbation   Masturbation means feeling the genitals to give oneself sexual pleasure. Many people believe that masturbation is evil or wrong. They feel guilty about doing it and want others to feel guilty as well. This is sad as masturbation is as natural as laughing. It is something anyone can do with their body which is enjoyable and does no harm to anyone else. Masturbation is only bad for a person if they believe it is — then they will worry and feel guilty.

Boys and girls, men and women, all masturbate. Even babies

45

masturbate, though they will not reach orgasm. They soon discover that touching some parts of the body feels extra good. If adults see children touching their genitals they may tell them not to, so that the child feels guilty. Obviously masturbating is like going to the toilet — it is something one does in private.

Teenagers usually masturbate more often than other age groups. Many adults masturbate if they have no partners, or if they want to have an orgasm on their own or they do not want to get pregnant. No woman has ever got pregnant by masturbating. And nobody has ever caught a sexually transmitted disease by masturbating. Married people masturbate too, if their partner is away or does not feel like sexual intercourse. Sometimes they help masturbate each other. Masturbating is a way of understanding how your body works and feels.

Boys and men masturbate by stroking or rubbing the penis backwards and forwards in their hands until they ejaculate. They may put cream or oil on the penis to make it slippery.

Girls and women masturbate by stroking or rubbing the vulva, clitoris and vagina with their fingers until they reach orgasm.

Masturbation can take anything from a few minutes to an hour. This depends on the mood of the person and how much time they have.

While masturbating many people imagine they are with someone they know, or with someone they would like to know, such as a film star. They may imagine doing things that are normally unacceptable or impossible such as making love on a motorbike

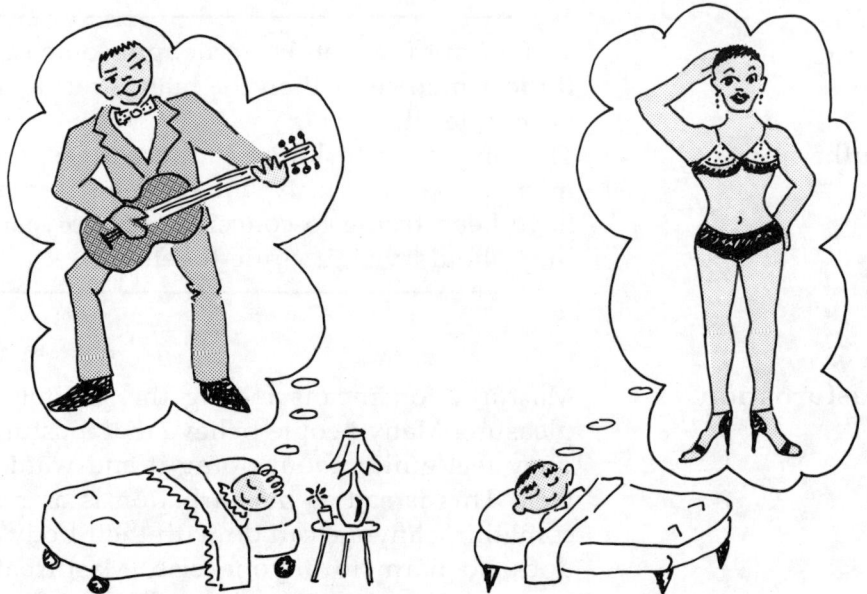

Everyone has fantasies.

in the market! Everyone has fantasies, especially if they have read a book or seen a film in which the hero or heroine always gets the most beautiful partners!

One cannot masturbate 'too much', but sometimes people with problems find they masturbate more often. This may help them forget their problems for a short time, but it will not help them solve their problems. Anyone with problems will find they are solved better by talking to their parents, a teacher or an older friend than by masturbating.

Some people think of masturbation as a poor substitute for sexual intercourse with someone. It is different and can be just as pleasurable and certainly relieves tension.

Not everyone feels like masturbating, but if they do they should not feel bad about it, as it does no harm.

Dear Auntie,

I read somewhere that masturbating makes you go blind. I have enjoyed masturbating for three years. Will I really go blind?

Peter

Dear Peter,

You cannot go blind from masturbating. It does no harm to the body or to the mind. Other myths about masturbating include the idea that the penis will drop off, or you will become infertile, go mad, ruin your marriage, grow warts, use up all your semen or get terrible acne. Of course, someone with acne may have masturbated. But this does not mean that masturbation caused the acne!

The only harm is if you feel bad about it, or you are not gentle with yourself or masturbate using sharp or dangerous instruments.

Infertility

Many couples find that the woman cannot get pregnant when they want a baby. If the woman is not pregnant after two years, then the man or woman may be **infertile**, or **sterile**. In half the cases it is the man who is infertile. People used to think it was always the woman who was infertile. The couple should visit a doctor together. The doctor will carry out tests on both the man and the woman.

The man will be asked to ejaculate some semen into a jar. This is looked at under a microscope to count the sperm in the semen. The man may produce semen, but with only a few sperm in it. A low sperm count is a common reason for male infertility. If a husband makes only a few sperm at each ejaculation then several samples of his semen can be collected and stored at the clinic. The sperm are then mixed together and put inside the woman all at once when she is ovulating. Although only one sperm is needed for fertilization, so many sperms die on the way to the ovum, that many million are needed to ensure that fertilization takes place.

If the man produces no sperm, then the woman can have some sperm from another man put inside her. She does not have sexual intercourse with the man — she never meets him. This is called **artificial insemination**, or A.I. The couple bring up the baby as if they were both natural parents.

In a woman the ovaries or the fallopian tubes may have been damaged by disease. This prevents the sperm reaching the ovum. Many infertile women have periods, but produce no ovum. Blood tests can show if ovulation is happening. Other woman may get pregnant, but the embryo will not grow in the uterus and keeps coming out as a late menstrual period or a **miscarriage**.

Infertility in a woman can often be cured with a small operation or by taking special drugs. Infertility in a man is more difficult to cure.

A couple may be making love at the wrong time of the month for conception to occur. The fertility clinic can explain to the couple the best time to have sex to achieve pregnancy (see Chapter 5, page 95).

Some people are born infertile. Many others become infertile from infections which block up the tubes carrying the sperm or the ova.

Although doctors cannot cure every infertile couple, they can help many. Traditional healers or medicine cannot cure infertility and may make it worse.

If the couple are told by the doctor that they cannot have children then it is not the end of the world. They can still lead happy and fulfilled lives.

Adoption or fostering orphaned babies is as satisfying as being natural parents. Adoptive parents can love their children just as much as natural parents. And they know they are helping a child who would otherwise have no home or family. Many couples adopt children when they have had one or two of their own.

Some infertile couples decide that without children they can concentrate on their careers or helping other people. There are many ways of leading a fulfilling life without being parents.

Rape

Rape means a man forcing a woman to have sexual intercourse against her will. Men can rape women, but women cannot rape men. Husbands can rape their wives, but this may not be illegal. However, marriage does not excuse rape. In some countries men can be hanged or shot for rape.

Many cases of rape are not reported to the police, because the woman is ashamed. Proving that a man has raped a woman can be difficult. The rapist may say, 'I thought that when she said "No" she really meant "Yes".' The rapist is usually known by the woman. This makes proof of rape even more difficult. The rapist may say that the woman was immoral so it did not matter.

Every man who has raped a woman is mentally sick. Any man who feels like raping a woman should remember that women are people with feelings, and not bodies to be used for sex. Alcohol makes some men violent. The same men who fight men when they are drunk, may rape women. Some men think that women enjoy being raped. Rape is always frightening, and a violent act against a woman. Many women take years to recover from rape and are afraid of all men afterwards. They need reassurance, love, healing and patience.

Women can help to protect themselves from rape. Never walk alone late at night. If you have to walk home alone, use a street with lots of people. Avoid the streets with lots of bars. Do not walk along empty roads. Do not accept lifts from men in cars. If you have to walk alone, walk as fast as possible – do not look around you or look at any men. Carry an umbrella or walking stick you can use as a weapon if necessary.

If you think a man is going to rape you, try to stay as calm as possible, even if the man has a knife or gun. Screaming loudly may make him run away if you are outdoors. While you are still standing up, try and kick him in the testicles with your knee. You must do this very hard to stop him. If you hit him gently, he will get more angry and excited. If he gets you on the ground, remember what the man looks like. Tell him that you do not want sex. Sometimes talking calmly to a man will make him go away. The important point is not to get hurt and to show him you do not want sex. The more you struggle, the more he may hurt you, or get more excited.

When the man has gone away get help quickly. Find a friend or relation and tell them exactly what happened, as you may need a witness.

Some women are more afraid of the questioning by the police after the rape than they were of the rape, so they do not report it. If you decide to tell the police then do so as soon as possible. Do not wash, or tidy yourself, or change your clothes. Do not have a bath because the semen from the rapist can be used as evidence against him in court. Do not drink any alcohol. Go to the police with your friend. The police may ask you many difficult questions. The police will need a medical examination. Ask them for a woman doctor and for your friend to remain with you. Take a change of clothes with you, as the police may want to keep your clothes as evidence against the rapist.

In some countries the newspapers are not allowed to print the names of women who are raped. In other countries they can, so the woman may not want to report the rape because it may appear in the newspapers.

Even if you decide not to report the rape to the police, find a friend and talk to them about it. Have a pregnancy test and a test for sexually transmitted diseases as soon as possible.

Homosexuality

Some men are sexually attracted to other men, and some women desire other women. Probably about four per cent of people are **homosexual, lesbian** or **gay**. In many countries this does not appear because men and women are frightened to admit it. You cannot tell if someone is homosexual by looking at them.

Homosexuals give pleasure to each other just like **heterosexuals** – kissing, laughing, stroking and talking. If the couple are happy about it, homosexuality does no harm to anyone else. Some, though not all, male homosexuals have **anal intercourse**. This can spread **AIDs** (see Chapter 6, page 132).

In many countries it is illegal for two people of the same sex to make love. In some countries it is illegal for men, but not for women. Most countries have a strong taboo against homosexuality. Homosexuals may find it difficult to get jobs, or make friends.

No-one knows why some people are homosexual. It may be hormones, or an influence in their childhood. Homosexuality is not a disease. It cannot be caught, and it cannot be cured. Trying to cure homosexuals with drugs, or in mental hospitals will only make them confused and depressed.

Young people may feel confused if they are attracted to friends of the same sex. Discussing this with an understanding adult can help. For many the feeling fades away as they find making friends of the opposite sex easier.

Some people are physically attracted to friends of both sexes. This is called being *bisexual*.

Many people are frightened of homosexuals and think they want to chase young children. Homosexuals are no more likely to attack children than heterosexuals. Homosexuals are not attracted to every person of their sex. They are the same as heterosexuals: they like some people and do not like others.

Homosexuals cannot have babies or get married. But they can

have lasting and loving relationships just like any married couple. They are ordinary people who can contribute as much to society as anyone else. A homosexual can be a shop keeper, a bank clerk, a teacher or a nurse. Whether homosexual, bisexual or heterosexual, everyone should be accepted by their families and society as people, with human feelings.

Activities

1 Each person in the group writes down a sentence that men use to persuade women to have sex with them. For example, 'You might as well do it − I shall tell everyone you did anyway'; 'This is the way to prove you really love me'; 'It is your fault that I am all excited. Now you must do something about it'; or 'You are the only one I've ever asked'. Then the group thinks of replies they could say to these remarks. This helps young women to have the confidence to say 'No' and shows young men that they cannot control women.

2 Discuss different activities which young men and women can do together which will not lead on to sex. Make up a role play about young men and women going out together and the different ways they can behave towards each other.

3 Women − practice the exercises on page 24 which help relieve painful periods.

4 Women − is there a 'Judith Club' in your area? These are clubs for teenage women which help to equip them for the pressures of modern society, including sexual pressures from men. The members are taught confidence, motivation and tactics for handling men trying to put sexual pressure on them. They learn about the benefits to themselves, their bodies and their future children of not sleeping around. Judith is in the Old Testament of The Bible. She was very wise, with courage and intelligence, knowledge of how men think and feminine charm. Members of Judith Clubs do not have to be Christians. Young women can also learn other knowledge and skills necessary for adult life, such as nutrition and child care.

CHAPTER 4
Pregnancy and birth

Pregnancy

The fertilized ovum travels from the fallopian tube to the uterus. Pregnancy starts at **conception** when the new **embryo** arrives in the uterus about a week after fertilization. The lining of the uterus is soft and full of blood vessels, ready to nourish the embryo. The embryo settles into the lining and the cells begin to multiply, each section growing into a different part of the body

Placenta

Within a few days a **placenta** forms out of the embryo. The placenta is attached to the lining of the uterus rather like a plant's roots growing in soil. They are together, but different. The placenta is part of the baby, not part of the mother. As the baby grows, so the placenta grows to nourish it with food and air from the mother's blood. Every baby has its own placenta.

The placenta is attached to the baby by a tube called the **umbilical cord**. This grows from the middle of the placenta to the centre of the baby's abdomen. The **navel** is where the umbilical cord entered our bodies before we were born. The umbilical cord is a two way tube of blood vessels. It is up to 50 cm long when the baby is born.

In the placenta the baby's blood flows past the mother's blood and picks up a new supply of food and **oxygen**. All the food that the growing baby needs comes through the placenta and umbilical cord. The heart of the baby pumps the blood along the umbilical cord and around its body. The baby's blood and the mother's blood do not mix, but they flow so close together that food and air can pass between them. This 'food' is not like a meal on a plate — it is already digested by the mother. If the mother eats well then the baby will be fed well.

The placenta is also a filter. Many harmful products that are in the mother's blood are stopped from reaching the baby. But it cannot filter out all harmful materials. Some diseases and some drugs can pass from the mother to the baby. Certain diseases can cause the baby to be born deformed. **Rubella** (German measles) is a contagious disease which is not dangerous to adults. But if a mother has rubella in the first three months of pregnancy the baby may be born deaf, blind or brain damaged.

Medicines that may be good for adults can be dangerous to unborn babies. Some medicines cause small, weak babies, others can cause the babies to be born **deformed**, such as with no legs. Not all medicines have been tested properly to find out what harm they may do. So the safest course is not to take any medicines during pregnancy. Traditional herbal medicines can cause the baby to be born dead, or make the mother bleed heavily.

The **nicotine** from cigarettes causes many babies to be born small and weak. Babies of women who smoke are on average 200 gm lighter than other babies. Pregnant women should not smoke cigarettes, or pipes. If both parents smoke then it is much easier for the mother to stop smoking if the father does too. (See Chapter 7, page 157.) If both parents stop smoking they will feel healthier, live longer and have a healthy baby.

Smoking is bad for babies, and mothers.

Alcohol also passes to the baby from the mother and can cause small, weak babies. A small drink is not harmful, but enough alcohol to make a mother drunk may harm the baby. Babies born to mothers who drink a lot often have problems with breathing and suckling.

Uterus

The uterus is a bag of muscle, normally the size of a chicken's egg. As the baby and placenta grow the uterus grows too. After six weeks of pregnancy the uterus has grown to the size of an orange. The uterus holds the baby and placenta safely and also pushes them out at birth. A pregnant woman's **abdomen** feels hard and tight. The uterus is made of strong muscles, like a footballer's legs. Giving birth is far more hard work for the uterus and the mother than any football game!

The **cervix** at the base of the uterus stays tightly closed during pregnancy to hold the baby in.

The baby floats in water which protects it from any knocks the mother may have. The water allows the baby to move about inside the uterus. By five months the mother can feel her baby kicking and waving its arms. The baby can even turn right over. The baby swallows the water and it passes through its body and goes in and out of the baby's lungs. The baby is not eating or breathing but the water makes sure that the intestines and lungs are working. During the birth the water helps the baby to come out.

From about 24 weeks the baby has everything a human needs

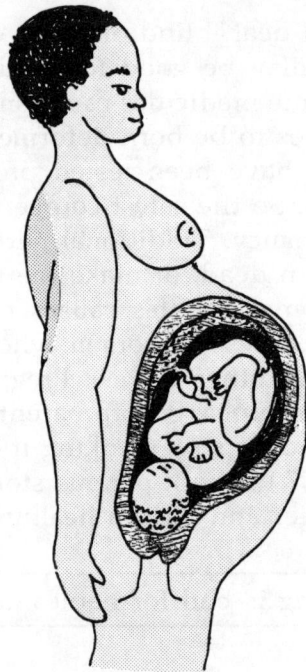

The baby's position at 9 months.

to live. But the baby is very small and the breathing muscles have not developed. The layer of fat under the skin has not grown so the baby loses heat very quickly. A tiny baby cannot adapt to different temperatures and will stop breathing if cold.

From 32 weeks the baby could live, but only with very special care. **Premature** babies are so small that they need frequent feeding and extra warmth.

By the eighth month the baby's head is pointing downwards into the mother's pelvis. At 40 weeks the baby is ready to be born, and strong enough to cope with the journey to the outside world.

First signs of pregnancy

- One or more missed periods.
- Swollen, tender breasts.
- Nausea — feeling sick, especially in the morning.
- Tiredness.
- Need to urinate often.

Dangers of smoking in pregnancy

- Greater risk of problems during the birth.
- High risk of premature birth.
- Nicotine is passed into baby's blood. Among other things, this makes the baby's heart beat too fast.

- **Carbon monoxide** passes from the cigarettes into mother's blood. The baby gets less oxygen and does not grow well.
- Higher risk that baby will be small. Smaller babies are weaker babies.

Growth of baby in the uterus

Age	Average size	Development
2 weeks	1.5 mm	Embryo settles into the uterus. Already male or female. Placenta growing.
3 weeks	3 mm	The size of this 'E'. Heart and eyes forming.
5 weeks	1 cm	Brain and backbone forming. Arms and legs are small 'buds.'
6 weeks	1.5 cm	The size of a peanut. Heart begins to beat.
8 weeks	2.5 cm	Eyes formed, but no eyelids. Hands and feet growing.

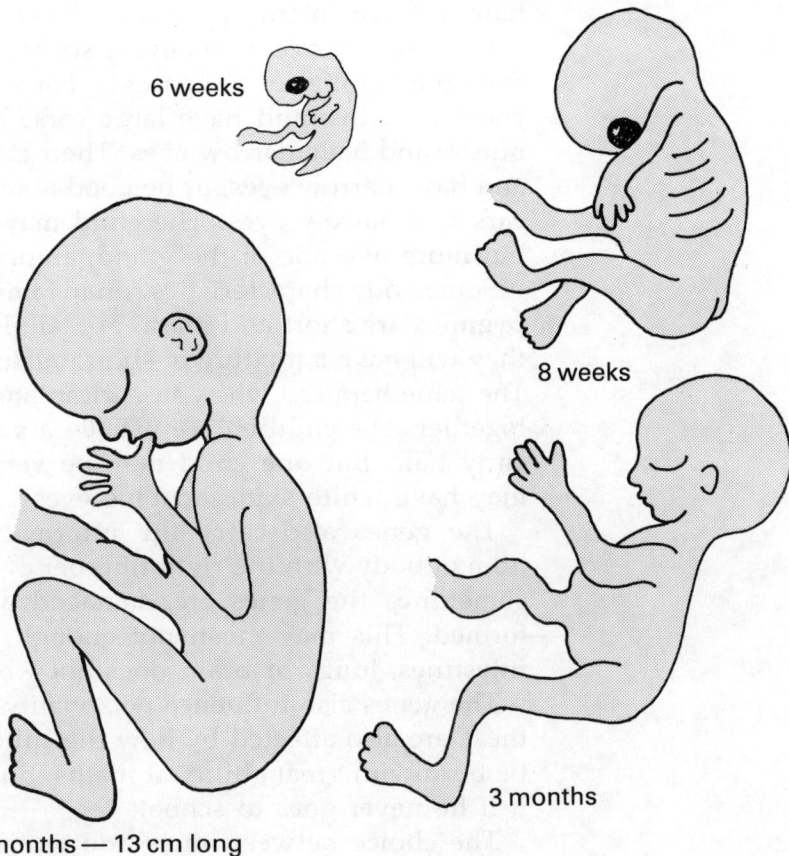

6 weeks

8 weeks

3 months

4 months — 13 cm long

Stages of embryo growth.

Age	Average size	Development
3 months	6 cm	Looks like a human baby with features of face and genitals.
4 months	13 cm	Begins to move around. Hair grows on head and body. Fingernails grow. Hands and feet have individual fingerprints.
5 months	16 cm	Mother feels movement. Baby may suck thumb.
6 months	24 cm	If born now, can sometimes live. Eyes open and close. Swallows water. Loud noises make baby jump.
7 months	1.5 kg	Many babies born now will live. Baby is head down.
9 months	3 kg 50 cm	Ready to be born.

Genes

Each embryo contains about 100 000 genes, half from each parent. The parent's genes join and decide the baby's height and build, hair and eye colour.

Inside every ovum and every sperm are different characteristics from the families of the parents. For example, the mother may be good at maths, and have large ears. The father may be good at music, and have narrow eyes. Their child could be good at maths and have narrow eyes, or be good at maths, music and have large ears and narrow eyes. The child may not be like either parent, but more like one of the grandparents!

Some body characteristics run in families, or tribes. For example, **pygmies** are short and **masai** are tall. If a pygmy marries a masai they will have a mixture of short, tall and medium sized children. The same happens when an African and a European have children together. The children are usually a pale brown colour, with soft curly hair. But one child may be very black and another child may have white skin and blue eyes.

The genes also carry the information for making a normal human body with the right number of arms, fingers and toes. But sometimes the genes are damaged and the baby is born deformed. This may mean not enough fingers or that the baby's intestines, lungs or brain does not work well.

The genes also influence personality and intelligence, although these are also affected by how the child is cared for. A child may be born with great ability at maths, but he will not be able to use it if he never goes to school.

The choice between male and female is made by the father's genes. Neither the father nor the mother can influence what sex their child will be.

Ante-natal clinic

Ante-natal clinics help to save the lives of many mothers. They help them to deliver healthy babies. In most countries ante-natal clinics are free. If a mother has to pay for each visit, she is spending her money wisely.

At the clinic the mother can ask the nurse questions about her pregnancy, the birth or the baby. The nurse is there to help. Pregnancy and birth are easier if the mother understands them.

If the mother takes any medicines given by a clinic she should tell the nurse. Medicines or herbs which are not from a clinic should not be taken by pregnant women.

During pregnancy there is a greater risk of **malaria**. Malaria can cause miscarriages or premature births, as well as being a dangerous disease for the mother. All pregnant women should take tablets provided by the clinic to prevent malaria.

On a first visit to an ante-natal clinic this is what will happen.
● Previous pregnancies, births and diseases, and health of the family will be discussed.
● The place of birth will be decided. If this is the second pregnancy and everything went well last time, then home is usually the best place. But if there were problems before, or there may be problems this time, then delivering the baby in a hospital or clinic is safer. Some mothers are 'at risk'. This means the birth should go well, but something might go wrong. If problems occur, then hospitals have nurses and doctors and the right equipment to save the baby's or the mother's life.

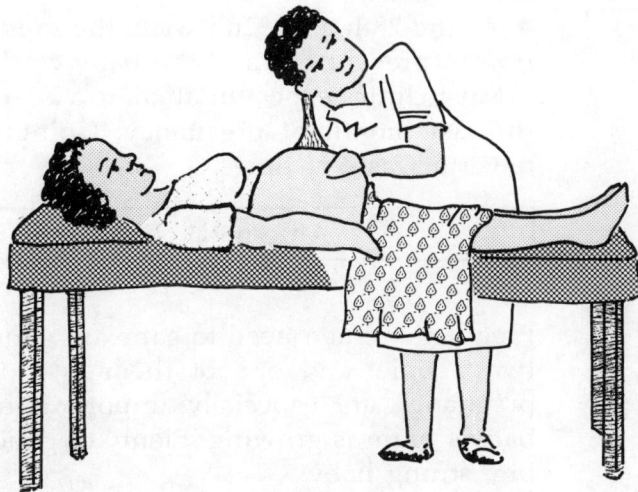

An ante-natal clinic.

Some births are so quick that the baby is born at home. These are often the easiest births.

Some hospitals and clinics have special houses for women waiting to be mothers. Women who live far away can come and stay for the last few weeks of their pregnancies. They can rest from work and eat a good diet. This helps the baby to grow and the mother remains strong.

If the mother chooses to deliver her baby at home, then she must find a good **midwife** to help her. The midwife should be trained in delivering babies. She should be able to recognise possible problems and take the mother to hospital if necessary.

• The nurse will work out the date the baby is expected using the date of the mother's last period. So it helps if she can remember the date.

*• The nurse will also weigh the mother, test her blood and urine and check her feet and hands for swelling. She will measure the **blood pressure** with a rubber tube wrapped around the upper arm. The nurse will listen to the blood passing through the arm. This is quite painless. If blood pressure is too high then problems can occur later. A pregnant woman can make her blood pressure low by resting often. Sometimes the blood pressure is so high that a mother must rest in hospital.

*• The abdomen will be felt to check baby's growth and position. From about five months the nurse can use a special instrument to hear the baby's heart beat.

• At each visit the nurse will do all above marked * and also give a talk or lesson on pregnancy, diet, breastfeeding or baby care. This gives mothers a chance to learn, and talk about their worries or problems.

• At the 28th and 32nd week the mother will be given an injection to prevent her and the baby catching **tetanus**.

Most clinics expect mothers to visit once a month and twice in the last month of pregnancy. Going to an ante-natal clinic is never a waste of time.

Ante-natal clinics save many lives.

Food

Pregnant women need to eat extra good food as they are feeding two people, and one of them is growing! The last weeks of pregnancy are especially important because this is when the baby's brain is growing. Plenty of good food will help to make a big, strong baby.

Everyone, especially a pregnant mother, needs a mixture of good foods, or a **balanced diet**. Try and eat a mixture of different foods every day.

Good food — eat as much of these as possible	_Vegetables_	_Fruit_	_Dairy foods_
	Pumpkin	Avocado pears	Milk
	Green beans	Oranges	Sour milk
	Peas	Lemons	Cheese
	Cabbage	Grapefruit	
	Carrots	Grapes	
	Onion	Pineapples	
	Tomatoes	Mangoes	
	Spinach	Guavas	
	Okra	Bananas	
	Sweet potatoes		
	Wild green leaves		
	Green maize		

Meat, fish, eggs, insects, such as flying ants and caterpillars, shellfish, millet, sorghum, sesame, lentils, beans, nuts, peanut butter.

Eat enough of these   Margarine, cooking oil, cassava, plantains, unrefined maize meal, brown bread, brown rice. Brown flour and unrefined meal prevent constipation.

Do not eat too many of these foods —   they will not help your baby grow. Sweets, biscuits, fizzy drinks, beer, sugar, cakes, wine, chocolate.

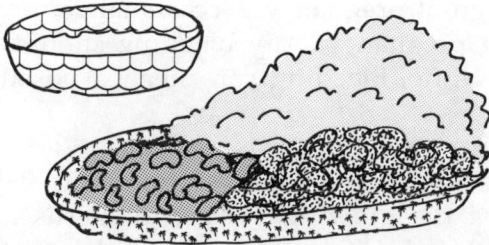

Milk curds, maize porridge, beans and cabbage

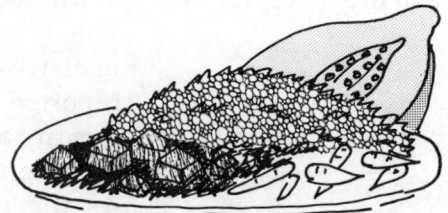

Rice carrots, meat and paw-paw

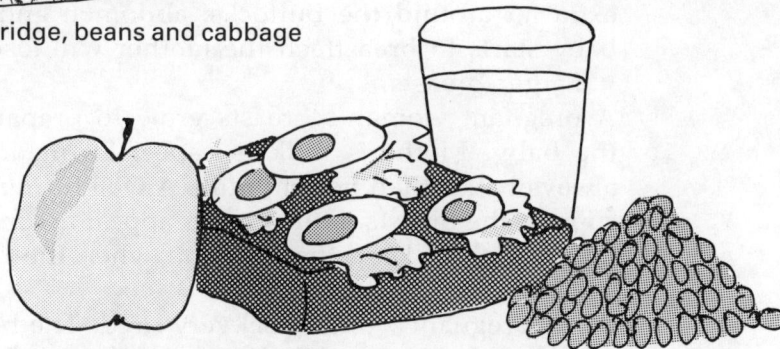

Egg, spinach, bread, nuts, milk and apple

Good foods to eat in pregnancy.

59

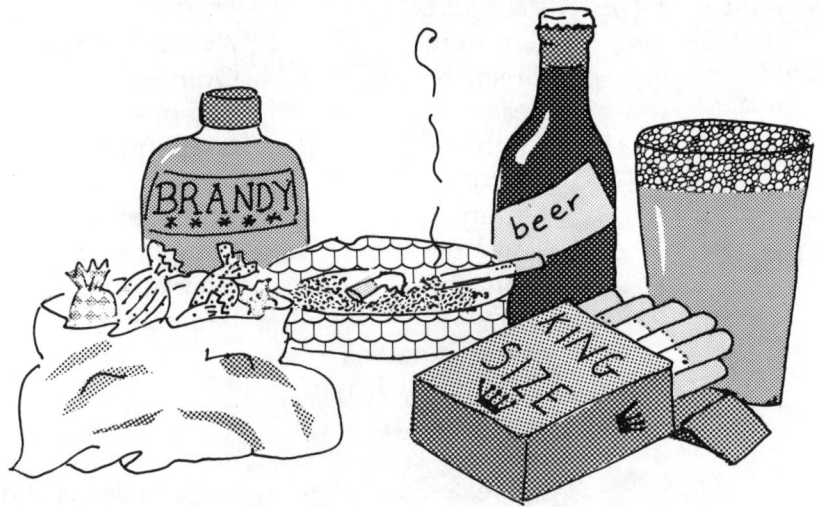

Things to avoid in pregnancy.

Clothes

Loose, cotton dresses are more comfortable to wear. Dresses that unbutton down the front can also be worn later when breast-feeding the baby. Flat shoes or bare feet put less strain on the back and legs than high heels.

Body changes during pregnancy

Not all these changes happen to every woman.
● Missed periods
This is normally the first sign of pregnancy. Occasionally a pregnant woman bleeds during pregnancy. Any bleeding should be reported to the ante-natal clinic. Bleeding can mean a possible miscarriage.
● Weight gain
As the pregnancy advances all women grow fatter. This extra weight is a combination of the growing baby and uterus and extra fat around the buttocks, abdomen and breasts. When the baby starts to breastfeed the mother will lose the extra weight.
● Larger breasts
A pregnant woman's breasts grow to prepare to make milk for the baby. Mother's milk is especially made for babies and is always better than bought milk. A well fitting cotton bra will help support the breasts. Little bumps appear around the nipples. These produce oil to keep the skin soft when the baby sucks.
● Tiredness
Many pregnant women feel very tired. The body needs plenty of rest and sleep. The whole family must help with the work — especially heavy jobs. Sometimes tiredness is due to anaemia, or weak blood. The clinic can prescribe iron tablets, which are safe

for the mother and baby. Eating green vegetables strengthens the blood.

● Nausea

Most pregnant women feel sick during the first three months. The nausea is often worse in the morning and may lead to vomiting. Eating some bread or biscuits before getting up can help. Ask someone to bring you a cup of tea in bed. Lots of small meals rather than one or two big meals can reduce the nausea.

Do not take any medicines to stop the nausea. Early pregnancy is the most dangerous for medicines. Many babies have been born deformed after their mothers took medicines to relieve nausea and vomiting. Although unpleasant, it is better to bear it. By three months the nausea has usually stopped.

● Indigestion

During the last few weeks the baby presses on the mother's stomach which can cause indigestion. Drinking milk and eating small meals often helps. Certain foods such as hot curries and fatty meat can increase indigestion.

● Constipation

Taking medicines or herbs for constipation could harm the baby. Drink extra water and eat lots of fresh fruit and vegetables and brown bread.

● Cramp in the legs

This can be helped by rubbing the legs or taking exercise.

● Breathlessness

During the last few weeks the baby may press on the lungs and make you short of breath, especially when lying down. Sleep with lots of pillows.

● Need to urinate

The baby starts to press against the bladder when it is still very small. A pregnant woman should not drink less so that she needs to go to the toilet less often. She should drink even more, and go to the toilet often.

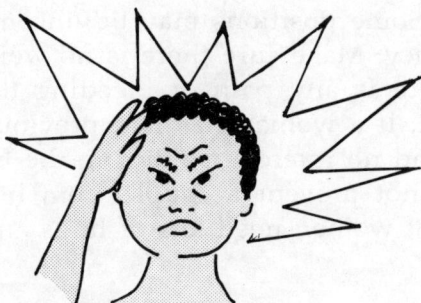

Bad headaches   Swollen ankles

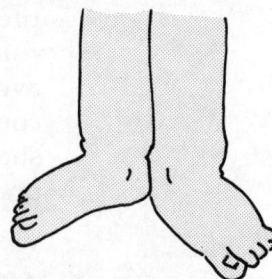

Danger signs in pregnancy.

These could become dangerous if not treated at a clinic.
- Swollen ankles or hands

These are a sign that the mother should rest more. Lie down with your feet higher than your body as often as possible every day.
- Headaches

Bad headaches should be reported quickly to the ante-natal clinic or a doctor. They may be a sign of high blood pressure.
- High blood pressure

A woman cannot know if she has high blood pressure without going to the clinic. But if she has it, then she must take extra rest as high blood pressure is a danger to the baby and the mother.

Feelings

Pregnancy should be a happy time of looking forward to the new baby. But many women feel confused. For no reason they cry or feel angry at nothing. The husband and the family need to have extra understanding and sympathy. There is the worry about how she will cope with the baby and whether the birth will go well and the baby will be normal.

Fathers, too, may feel confused or worried. Fathers should be involved at all stages. If they are willing, they can go to the ante-natal clinic. The more a father knows about pregnancy and birth the more understanding and helpful he can be.

Other children in the family need reassurance about the new baby. Small children can become jealous of a new brother or sister if the baby gets all the attention.

If the pregnancy was not planned the woman may feel even more confused, worried or guilty. She may have practical problems such as not enough money or no man to support her. She will need even more support and sympathy from her family and friends. The mother and her baby will not be helped if she is told she is wicked and should not have got pregnant.

Sex in pregnancy

For most women sexual intercourse is quite safe during pregnancy. Some positions may be uncomfortable at the end of the pregnancy. Make sure there is no weight on the uterus.

If there is any pain or bleeding then intercourse should be avoided. If a woman has had previous miscarriages doctors recommend no intercourse during the first three months. But this should not prevent a couple from being close and loving. All pregnant women need lots of hugs and encouragement.

Birth

After 40 weeks the baby is ready to be born. Few babies are born on the exact date they are expected. They may be a few days early or a few days late.

The mother knows the baby is coming when she feels the uterus beginning to tighten. Or the water the baby is floating in may start to trickle out. The mother goes to the hospital or clinic, or she calls the midwife to her home. Everything should be clean and ready in her home. The midwife will need hot water, soap and clean cloths. The baby will need clean clothes and a blanket.

Labour

The time from when the **contractions** begin, to when the baby is born is called **labour**, because it is hard work for the mother. The uterus is a bag of thick muscle. The muscles contract tightly for a few seconds, and then relax. Gradually the time of each contraction increases. The uterus does not contract continuously. As the birth gets nearer, the contractions get stronger. This is when labour can be painful. The pain is not so bad if the mother breathes slowly and keeps calm and relaxed. Some clinics and hospitals give the mother gas or injections to ease the pain. Rubbing the back or the abdomen very gently helps the pain.

First the cervix must stretch open. This is the thickest part of the uterus so it may take several hours to open and allow the baby's head into the vagina. When the cervix is open the mother feels a strong urge to push the baby out. She may have been walking gently around, sitting or lying down.

The mother can give birth in several positions. Some women like lying on their backs. Others prefer to squat, kneel or sit up

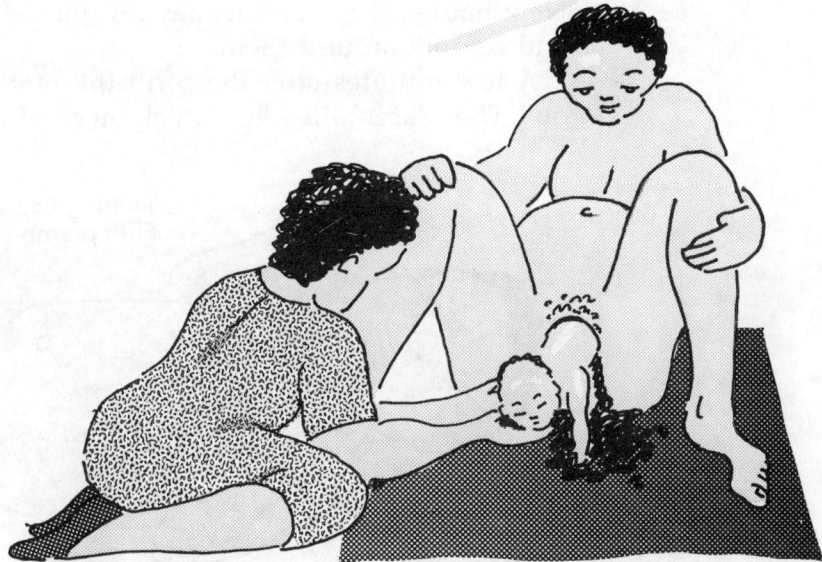

Birth.

with someone holding them behind. Birth is usually quicker and easier if the mother is standing or sitting upright.

The bag holding the water may burst before the birth or as the baby comes out. The baby is usually lying upside down with its head pointing downwards into the mother's pelvis. Birth is easier head first, though some babies are born feet first. The top of the head is slightly pointed and it stretches the birth passage. The parts of the skull slide over each other to make the head smaller. After pushing hard for 10 to 30 minutes the baby's head appears. A baby's head is wider than its shoulders, so the body slips out of the vagina easily after the head. The water helps the baby to come out smoothly.

Birth is different for every woman, and for each of her babies. For some mothers birth is quick and painless. For others it takes longer and is very tiring. Birth usually takes from 2 to 24 hours. The first birth usually takes longer than later births. A very long birth is not good for the baby.

As soon as they are born, babies start to breath and sometimes cry. The mother feels happy to have her baby at last, and quickly forgets about the birth pains. The skin of new born babies is often a strange purple-grey colour and not dark brown. Babies are covered in white cream which keeps the skin soft and protects it from germs. Their heads are out of shape and their faces screwed up. After a few days they become more beautiful! The baby is examined by the midwife. New babies have everything a person needs — fingers, eyes, ears, waving arms and legs and a loud voice — but they do not know how to use them yet. New babies can see, but they do not yet understand the shapes and colours around them.

A few minutes after the birth the mother pushes the placenta out. The placenta is like a thick piece of liver about 20 cm across

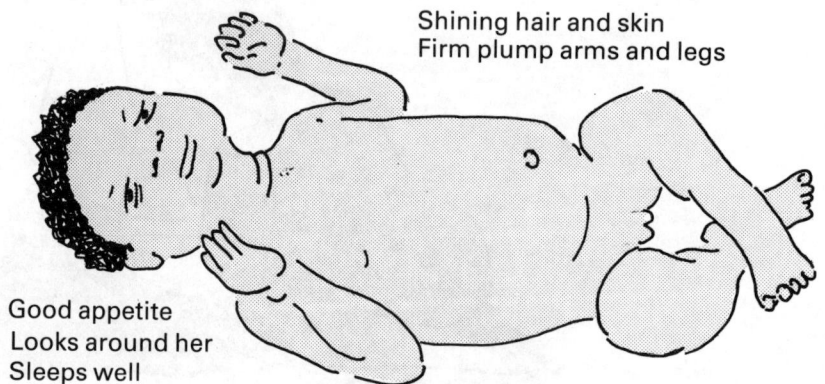

Shining hair and skin
Firm plump arms and legs

Good appetite
Looks around her
Sleeps well

A healthy newborn baby.

and 3 cm thick. The umbilical cord grows out of the centre. Wrapped around the placenta is the bag that held the baby and the water inside the uterus. It looks like a see-through plastic bag. These have done their work and so can be thrown away.

At birth the umbilical cord is attached to the baby's navel. It looks like a coiled wet rope. The cord is cut with a clean razor blade and tied to stop it bleeding. This does not hurt either the mother or the baby. The umbilical cord must be kept clean and dry. If mud or anything else is put on the cord then the baby may become very ill with tetanus. The umbilical cord dries up and drops off after a few days. It should never be pulled off. If there is any bleeding from the navel, or yellow **pus** then the baby should visit a clinic quickly.

For two or three weeks after the birth the mother will bleed as if she has a light period. Some mothers find that after the birth they have painful contractions for a few days, especially when the baby sucks the breast. This is because the sucking causes the uterus to contract to its normal size.

The baby is wrapped in warm clothes and given to the mother. Babies know how to breastfeed at once. Many babies have been sucking their thumbs already! The thick yellow milk produced by the mother for the first few days is very good for new born babies and should not be wasted. It gives the baby all the extra strength she needs to start her new life and helps protect the baby from diseases.

The mother is washed and may get up after a few hours rest. But she has worked hard to have her baby. She should only return to normal work when she feels well. She needs plenty of rest and good food to keep her strong and make milk for the baby.

Fathers can be very useful during the birth. They can give their wives support and comfort and enjoy the experience of seeing their baby's birth.

The mother should visit the ante-natal clinic after the birth with her baby. She should then take her baby to the Well Baby Clinic every month to be weighed and immunised against children's diseases.

Problems during birth

Occasionally the baby has difficulty in being born. The mother may have a small pelvis, or the birth may go on too long so the baby gets tired. The midwife may have to pull gently on the baby's head to help the baby out. This does not hurt the baby, though it may make the baby's head an odd shape for a day. A baby's head is not as hard as an adult's.

If the birth is very quick, or the baby is very large then the skin around the vagina may tear. The midwife can sew up the tear with special thread.

If the baby cannot be born through the vagina then the mother may need a **Caesarian operation**. The mother is put to sleep by a doctor and the baby is pulled out through a hole in her abdomen. The hole is sewn up and the mother feels nothing. She stays in hospital for about two weeks. If one baby has been born by Caesarian operation, then the mother must have her next babies in hospital in case a Caesarian birth is needed again.

Planning ahead

After the birth sexual intercourse can begin again when the woman feels like it. Women who have had difficult births or who needed stitches will take longer. Most women feel ready for intercourse after about six weeks, but earlier or later is also normal. The father should never force himself on his wife.

During this time fathers may be feeling lonely. Even if the mother does not feel like intercourse, she should lie with her husband and hug him.

Contraception should be used from one month after the birth. Although breastfeeding stops ovulation and periods in most women, it is not a reliable method of child spacing. (See Chapter 5, page 114.)

Dear Auntie,

My cousin told me that there is a way to find out whether a pregnant woman is having a boy or a girl. Is this true?

Sam

Dear Sam,

There are many ways of guessing if the baby is a boy or a girl. Some people guess from the shape of the mother's abdomen. Other people try hanging things over the abdomen and watch which way they swing. Half the guesses will be correct!

There is an expensive test that can only be done in large hospitals. The water surrounding the baby is tested to find out if the child is formed properly. The test also shows the sex of the baby, but should not be done just for this because the test may cause a miscarriage in a few women.

Dear Auntie,

I am pregnant and I want to do the best for my baby. I have always had a slim waist and medium sized breasts. My husband has always been proud of my figure, so I do not want to spoil it. A friend told me that breastfeeding makes a woman's breasts hang low and that once you've had a child you can never get your waist back. Should I bottle feed my baby to keep my figure?

Juno

Dear Juno,

No! Breastfeeding is the best thing for your baby, *and* for your figure. You should breastfeed the baby for at least two years. During pregnancy the breasts grow bigger. If you wear a good bra, then the fibres holding the breasts up will not stretch. Make sure it is not too tight or it will squeeze the **milk ducts**.

The sucking of the baby makes the uterus contract. Mothers of bottle fed babies take longer to get their waists slim again. Breastfeeding will help you to lose the extra weight you have put on around the waist and buttocks. While you are breastfeeding your breasts will remain larger, but you can be proud of the good start you are giving your baby.

Miscarriages

A miscarriage is when the baby is born too early to live. This can be during the first to seventh months of pregnancy. Miscarriages in the first three months are quite common. Usually there is something wrong with the baby. Some women do not know they are pregnant when they miscarry. They may bleed like a heavy period and have an aching abdomen. After three months a miscarriage is similar to a birth. A miscarriage can be as sad for a mother as the death of her baby after a nine month pregnancy. A miscarriage does not mean a woman is unable to get pregnant again.

Twins

Sometimes a woman gives birth to more than one baby at one time. Twins and triplets are more common in Africa than in other parts of the world. About one in fifty births is **multiple**. Different societies treat twins in different ways. In some areas twins are special and treated with respect. In other places twins used to be killed at birth because the people believed the twins had evil spirits and would bring bad luck.

There is not much room inside a woman for twins, or triplets.

67

These babies are usually small and need extra special care after birth.

There are two types of twins — **identical** and **non-identical**, or fraternal.

Non-identical twins

Normally the woman's ovary releases one ovum each month. If more than one is released at one time and they are both fertilized by different sperms then the woman will have non-identical twins, or even triplets. These twins can be both boys, both girls or one of each sex. They are similar to a brother and sister born at different times.

Identical twins

Identical twins come from the same ovum and the same sperm. During its early development the embryo may separate into two groups of cells, which will grow into two separate babies. Identical twins are always the same sex with the same genes. They look the same, though people who know them well learn their differences of character.

Disabled babies

Sadly some babies are born **disabled** or deformed. Some disabilities can be seen at once, such as a deformed leg. Other disabilities may not be noticed for some time, such as deafness or brain damage. Disabilities are usually not the fault of the father or the mother. Some disabilities are caused because the baby did not grow properly in the uterus. Brain damage can happen while a baby is being born if the birth is difficult. The parents need lots of comfort and support from their friends and families to accept the disabilities of their baby. Disabled children can do many things that other people can do, but they may take longer to learn. With lots of help and encouragement the child can often live a normal life. Some countries have special schools for blind, deaf or mentally disabled children. Many children are better living in their own villages or streets surrounded by their families and friends. Even a child with a damaged brain can learn simple tasks to look after himself and help the family.

Disabled children can bring much joy, happiness and love into a family. The birth of a disabled baby does not have to be a disaster for the parents. But the parents will need much patience and love to appreciate the blessings of their disabled baby.

What is the best age to have a baby?

The safest age for both the mother and baby is between 20 and 30 years of age. Younger or older mothers may have more problems during the pregnancy or the birth. Of course, thousands of mothers above or below these ages have easy births and healthy babies. But more healthy babies are born to mothers between 20 and 30 years than at other ages.

Among teenage women, miscarriages are more common and the baby is often born too early. Babies of teenage mothers are on average smaller and weaker. This may be because a young mother does not eat well. A teenager's body has not finished growing so her pelvis may be too narrow for the baby to get out easily. If she has to leave school early she will miss her education. She may not know about ante-natal clinics, and good nutrition. If she goes back to school after the birth the young mother has to find someone to look after the baby. If the father is also at school he has the difficult choice of giving up school − and losing his education − or staying at school but not earning any money to support his new family.

Many young women feel dissatisfied with being school girls. They think that by becoming mothers they will grow into adult women more quickly. Becoming a mother is not easy. A woman needs to be emotionally mature, physically mature and economically stable with a man or a family to support her.

Being a parent means learning to love children, accepting their demands and working for them for at least 15 years. During the first year motherhood is especially tiring and difficult.

The majority of teenage pregnancies are unplanned. This is very sad as every baby should be a wanted baby. Adult parents can usually find a way of looking after an unplanned baby. But it is always more difficult for teenage parents. Sometimes the parents of the teenage mother send her away from home. This makes life even more difficult for both her and the new baby.

Between 20 and 30 years is both the safest age for mother and baby, and also the time when both parents have the energy to cope with small children. Over the age of 30 years the risks of problems in pregnancy gradually increase. Conception may take longer as a woman gets older. By 40 years the ovum are not so fresh and there is a higher risk of having a disabled baby. Women should try and have all the babies they want before they are 35 years old.

Activities

1 This activity gives young people the chance to experience the continual responsibilities of looking after a baby, without actually having one! For one week each person has to take complete responsibility for a chicken's egg. The egg must be kept warm and given fresh air. If the egg is left for any time, it must be in the care of another responsible person, but only for a short time. Should the egg be broken it is replaced after a day of 'mourning'. Each person keeps a daily diary on the life of the egg. Not

everyone will act responsibly and take the activity seriously, but it can be interesting to discuss why at the end of the week. At the end of the week everyone gathers with their eggs and their diaries. They discuss the activity and what they learnt from it about the continual care needed by babies.

2   Each student writes a list of up to 12 things they enjoy doing, either every day or once a week. They do not have to show this list to anyone else. They cross out each activity they could not do with a baby. How many activities would have to stop? Share and discuss how the young people's lives would be affected by parenthood.

3   Draw a poster advising pregnant women to attend ante-natal clinics. Find out the time and place of the local ante-natal clinic. Include this information on the poster.

4   Make up a role-play about pregnant women discussing how they live while pregnant. Some women eat healthy food and attend ante-natal clinics, other women smoke and drink. Which is better for the baby?

5   Discuss the different places where babies can be born. What are the advantages and disadvantages of these places?

CHAPTER 5
Child spacing and contraception

Contraception

This means preventing the sperm and ovum from meeting. There are several different ways of doing this. A couple may have to try several methods until they find the one that suits them. A contraceptive only works if it is used correctly by the couple. A condom lying unused by the bed will not prevent pregnancy. The couple must remember to use a condom every time.

One reason why there are so many unwanted pregnancies is that both partners think that contraception is the other's responsibility. Pregnancy is the responsibility of *both* partners. Both partners make a baby, even though it is the woman who has the

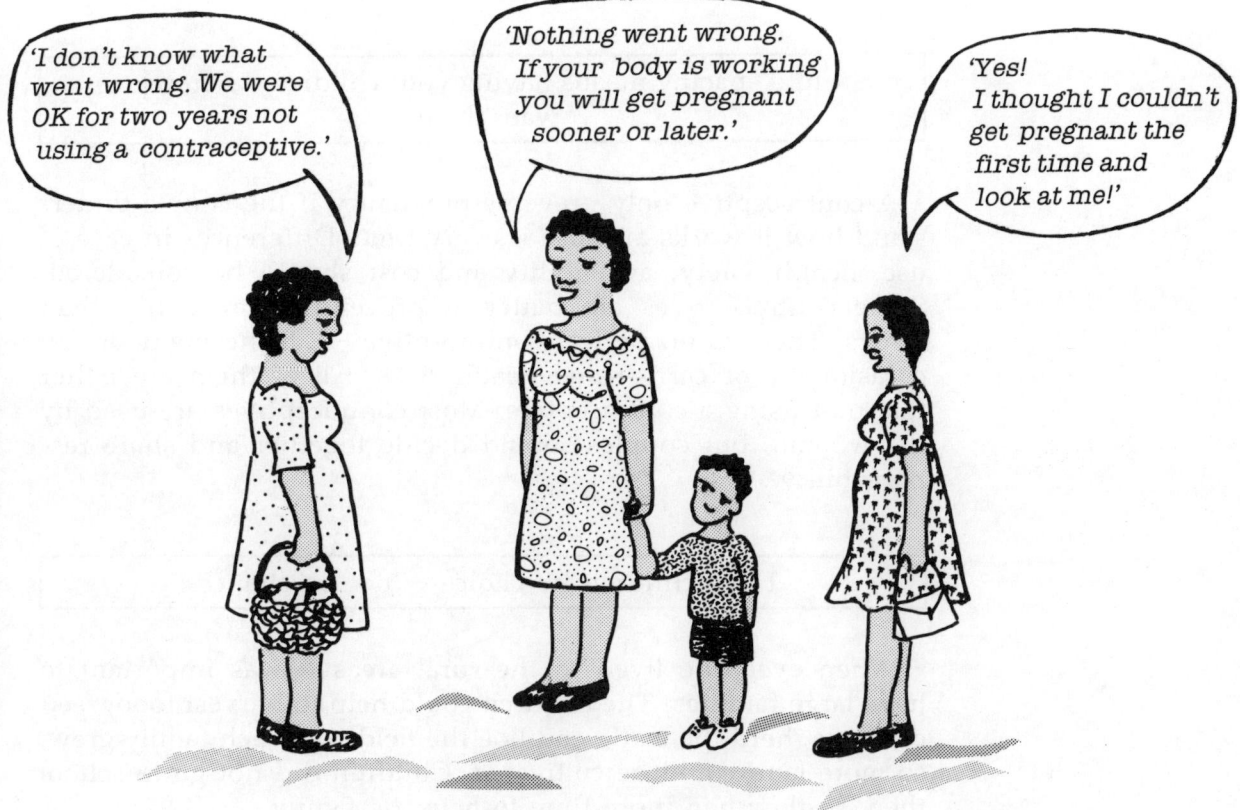

Do not ignore contraception

baby. Many women are embarrassed about using contraceptives because they might appear immoral. If a woman is willing to make love, than she must be willing to use contraceptives.

Many couples think that they are safe from pregnancy the first time they make love. The woman may be embarrassed to go to a clinic when she is a virgin. Some methods of contraception are not suitable for virgins but a man can use a condom, in this case.

The oldest and most reliable method of contraception is saying 'no'. No baby has ever been born after a woman said 'no' and the man accepted this.

Many couples still ignore contraception and just 'hope for the best'. If a couple do not like one method they should not say, 'We don't like contraceptives, we would rather take the risk of pregnancy'. They should return to their clinic and discuss other methods, or the woman will soon get pregnant.

Millions of babies are conceived by accident, even though there are several ways of preventing pregnancy. Nowadays every couple can choose when they want children. If a couple use contraception they can enjoy making love without the worry of an unwanted pregnancy. When a couple are ready to have children, their baby will be wanted and loved.

> Child spacing means having your children when you want them.

A contraceptive only prevents pregnancy if the couple understand how it works and use it every time. Differences in ease of use, health safety, availability and cost should be considered. Some contraceptives are better at preventing pregnancy than others. There is no perfect contraceptive — all the methods fail occasionally or carry some health risks. All of them are better than not using a contraceptive. Most contraceptives are used by the woman, but couples should decide together and share responsibility.

> Have children by choice — not by chance.

When everyone lived in the rural areas it was important to have large families. The children could help to harvest food, feed chickens, herd the cattle and hoe the fields. As each family grew, so more land could be cultivated. Children did not go to school then, so they had more time to help the family.

In the old days many more babies and children died young.

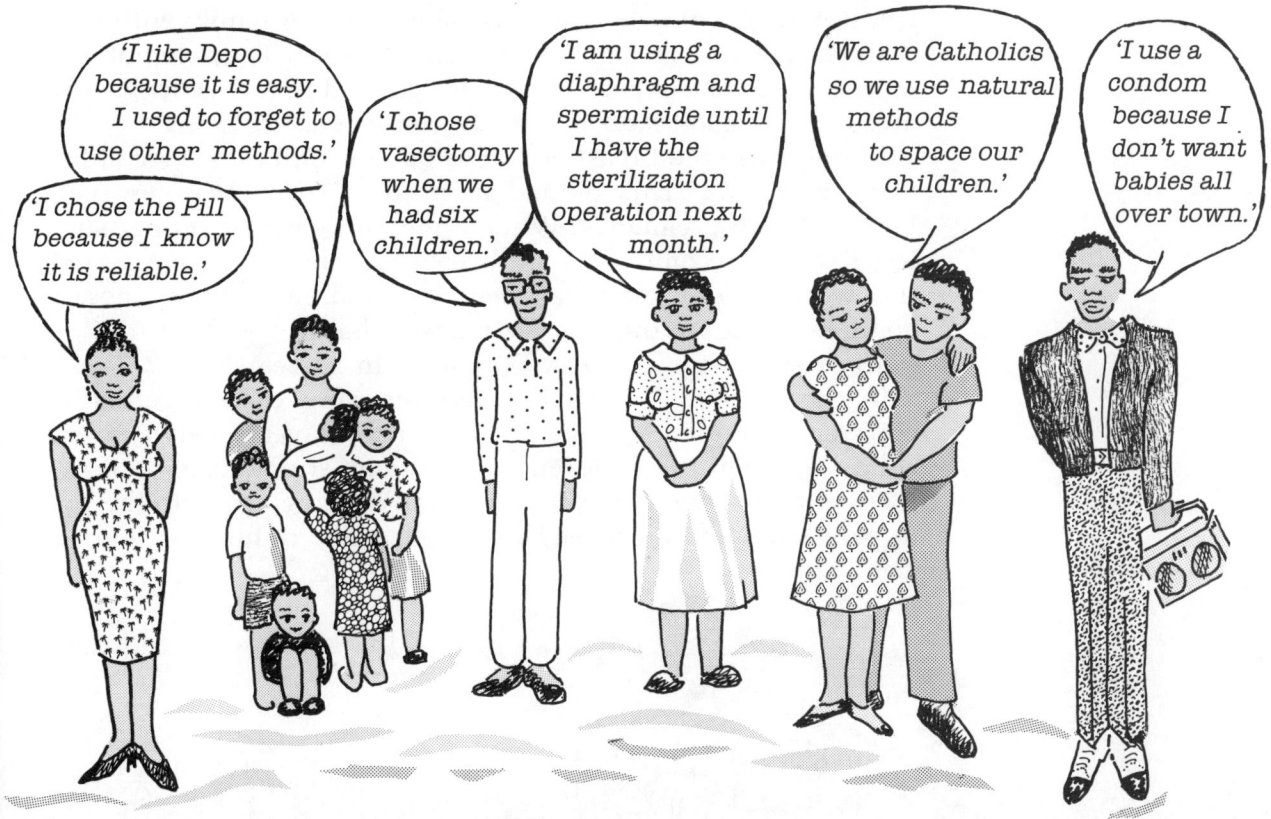

Different methods suit different people.

Sometimes whole families of children died in a few weeks from a disease such as measles. Parents had to have many children to make sure that some of their children survived to be adults. The mothers often died during pregnancy or childbirth. Or they were weakened and died young after having many babies close together.

Today everyone's health can be improved and most children live to be adults. If many babies are born, families will be bigger because most of them survive.

If everyone continues to have large families there will not be enough land or jobs for them all. There are already too many people for everyone to have as much land as they want, or the jobs they want.

A man earns the same amount of money whether he has two or twelve children. The mother has no time to work for money if she is busy looking after a large family. More children go to school nowadays, so they do not have time to cultivate land and help with small children. This means that mothers have even more work to do.

More people now live in towns and cities. A family with many children has to live together in a small house. They cannot grow more food because there is not enough land in towns. In the rural areas all the good land is already cultivated.

Mothers used to breastfeed their babies until they were at least three years old. This helped to make a space of a few years between each pregnancy. While a mother is breastfeeding she is less likely to become pregnant because she may not have periods. If a woman does not breastfeed her children and she does not space her children then she may have a baby every year until her periods stop. This could be 30 babies in 30 years!

If poor people have many children very close together the children may die. A space of at least three years between each child will keep the children and mothers strong. This will help them to overcome their poverty. Child spacing can help the poor to gain strength and to work for their basic rights.

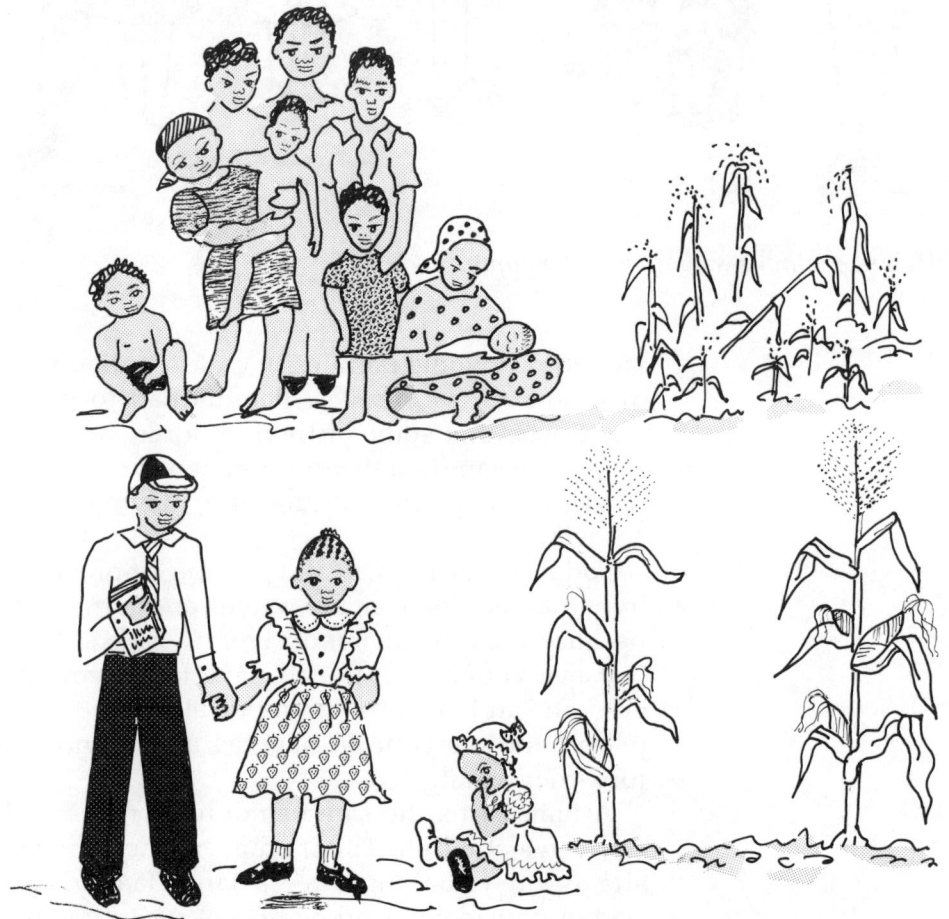

Children are like vegetables — they need space to grow.

Space between births

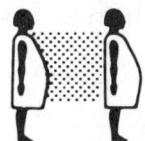

Less than 1 year — **200** Numbers of infant deaths (before age one) per 1000 live births.

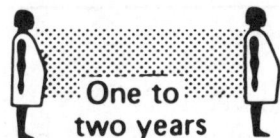

One to two years — **145**

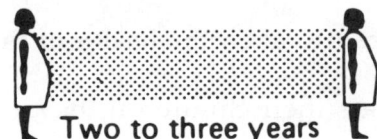

Two to three years — **100**

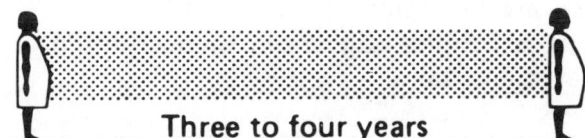

Three to four years — **80** Source: W.H.O. survey of 6000 women in South India.

Graph showing child spacing.

Child spacing

This means having a few years between the children in each family. A mother who has a new baby every year will have less time and energy to look after each child. If she waits three or four years she will be able to look after each baby well. The mother should breastfeed her child for at least two years. If the mother wants another baby after that, both of them will be strong. Mothers who have many babies in a short time may become sick and weak. A woman's body needs a rest between babies in order to regain strength.

If a woman is pregnant every year the babies are born smaller. Small babies are weaker and less healthy. If there is a longer space between children, then the children will be larger and healthier.

Having a baby every year is like growing many vegetables in a small patch of ground: all the vegetables will grow small and stunted. Some of them will die because each plant only has a small amount of food and water. If there is a big space between the vegetables they will each grow big and strong. Children are like vegetables: they need plenty of space between them. A space of three or four years between children is good. Then the parents can spend more time with each child. The children will have enough food, clothes and care. Fewer children in each family

75

means more food to share, so better health. There will be more money so better education. Well spaced children are stronger and do better at school.

> Well spaced children grow into strong healthy adults.

Advantages of child spacing

- Children have more food to eat.
- Children can be breastfed for at least two years.
- The first child has time with her mother before the next baby is born.
- Many pregnancies close together can weaken the health of the mother.
- Parents can feed, clothe and educate their children if they are well spaced.
- Well spaced children are healthier.

By using contraceptives couples can space their children and have babies when they want them.

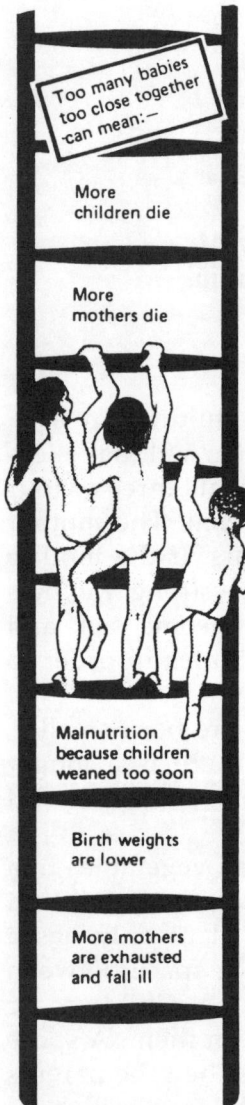

Too many babies too close together can mean:—

More children die

More mothers die

Malnutrition because children weaned too soon

Birth weights are lower

More mothers are exhausted and fall ill

Space for health

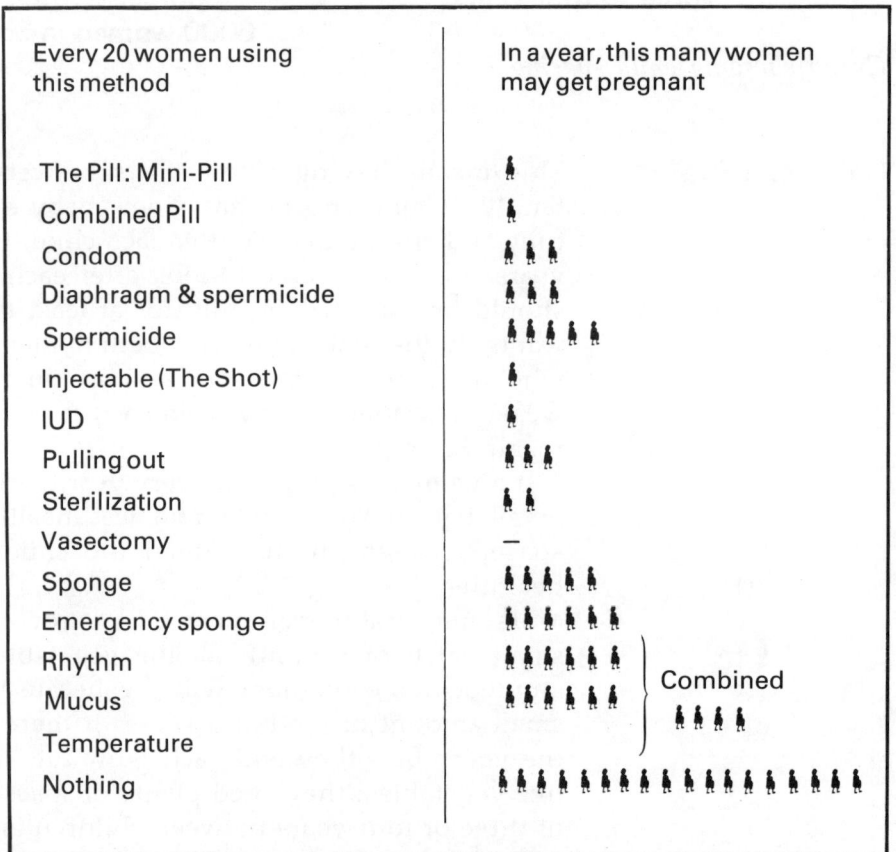

Every 20 women using this method	In a year, this many women may get pregnant
The Pill: Mini-Pill	♀
Combined Pill	♀
Condom	♀ ♀ ♀
Diaphragm & spermicide	♀ ♀ ♀
Spermicide	♀ ♀ ♀ ♀ ♀
Injectable (The Shot)	♀
IUD	♀
Pulling out	♀ ♀ ♀
Sterilization	♀ ♀
Vasectomy	—
Sponge	♀ ♀ ♀ ♀ ♀
Emergency sponge	♀ ♀ ♀ ♀ ♀ ♀
Rhythm	♀ ♀ ♀ ♀ ♀ ♀
Mucus	♀ ♀ ♀ ♀ ♀ ♀ } Combined ♀ ♀ ♀ ♀
Temperature	
Nothing	♀ ♀ ♀ ♀ ♀ ♀ ♀ ♀ ♀ ♀ ♀ ♀ ♀ ♀ ♀ ♀ ♀

Average protection of different contraceptives.

Are contraceptives safe?

Some methods of contraception may affect a woman's health. For example, women who smoke and are over 30 years should not use the Pill. The risk of ill health or death from unwanted pregnancy, however, is greater than the health risks of using contraceptives.

Contraceptives are safer than pregnancy.

Where to get child spacing advice

- Family planning clinics: good advice given; supplies of most methods; health check-ups.
- Hospitals: advice; sterilization operations; IUDs inserted.
- Doctors: advice and most methods supplied; health check-ups.
- Mother and child clinics: advice; most methods supplied; health check-ups.
- Village or community child spacing advisers: some advice; some methods supplied such as the Pill and condoms.
- Pharmacies: condoms; spermicides; diaphragms (or caps — woman must first be measured for correct size by a health worker).
- Barbers: condoms.
- Slot machines in toilets and beer halls: condoms, but may be out-of-date or poor brands.
- Markets: condoms; spermicides; the Pill, but may be out-of-date or wrong type.

Most governments want a healthy population of well-spaced families. In these countries contraceptive advice may be free or quite cheap. In some countries the governments want to increase the population so finding contraceptive advice can be difficult. Some religions do not approve of certain methods.

Some child spacing clinics only give advice to married couples. If you are having sex and you are not married then find a clinic or doctor who will give you advice. *Do not take risks*. Not all methods of contraception require a clinic or doctor. Anyone, man or woman, married or unmarried, can buy condoms and spermicide at pharmacies.

What happens at a child spacing clinic?

When a woman visits a child spacing clinic she will be asked by the nurse about her health, the size of her family and which contraceptive she may be using at the time. She will be asked about any diseases she has had. This is confidential — the clinic will not tell anyone else. The woman will be weighed and her blood pressure measured. Her breasts will be examined for unusual lumps (see Chapter 2, page 17). The nurse will explain the different methods of contraception. The woman should choose which she

77

thinks will be most suitable for her and her partner. Each method is suited to different couples.

If the woman chooses a cap the nurse will show her how to insert it. If she chooses an IUD then she may be asked to return to have it fitted.

The woman may be given a vaginal examination with a **smear** test. This is not painful. The nurse gently feels inside the vagina to find out if the uterus is in the right place. She then inserts a smooth metal instrument into the vagina and with a thin wooden stick she scrapes some of the mucus from the cervix. The cells in the mucus are then tested under a microscope to see if they are healthy.

The woman will be asked to return on a future date.

Men can also visit child spacing clinics. They may want to obtain condoms, or spermicides or to discuss a vasectomy operation. If a couple visit a child spacing clinic together then they can both learn about the different methods of contraception.

Some people know all about contraception, but they do not use it.

Why some people may not use contraception

- They are embarrassed or afraid to go to a clinic.
- They think that 'It won't happen to me. I can't get pregnant'.
- They feel that sex should just 'happen' and using contraception would ruin it.
- They do not want to admit to having sexual intercourse.
- They do not want to trouble their partners.
- They have heard stories from friends about the dangers of contraception.
- They have tried one method of contraception, but did not like it.
- They can't be bothered to go to a clinic or buy contraceptives.
- They feel that it is the other partner's responsibility.
- They have a deep-down desire to get pregnant to 'prove' their fertility.

These are all human reasons, but none of them are good enough reasons for not using contraception. The only reason for not using contraception is when a couple really want to have a baby.

Teenagers

As you read in Chapter 2, boys' and girls' bodies are ready to make babies when puberty begins. But they are not yet old enough for the difficult job of being parents. A girl can get pregnant when her periods start. But the pregnancy and birth could damage both the baby and herself. A school girl is not old enough to get married or to look after a baby well. A school boy is not old enough to be a good father and husband. Teenagers need to work hard at school or college so that they will be good parents when they grow up. Many girls and boys have to leave school because the girl gets pregnant. They have wasted the money of their parents. A school boy will find it difficult to get a job to support his young wife and baby. Only adults can cope with parenthood and marriage — and it is hard work even for them!

Some girls find school work hard. They think that if they have a baby their life will get better. It will not. Life is more difficult with a baby. Going to school will make her a better parent later on.

Teenagers cannot help falling in love. But they must remember that strong feelings can have serious results if they are not careful. Teenagers fall in and out of love very easily. Being in love does not mean that a couple have to make love. But if they do, they must use a contraceptive method. Some methods are not suitable for young people, because their bodies are still growing. The safest methods for young couples are the condom, or the Pill if periods are well established.

Dear Auntie,

My friends and I were talking about different methods of contraception. One girl said that some governments want to reduce the population by making us all infertile. Another girl said she had heard that they put contraceptive pills in school milk, so that we cannot have babies when we grow up. Is it safe to drink milk?

Emily

Dear Emily,

No government wants its people to be infertile. They want enough people in the country to make it wealthy. But many governments are worried about the high population increase and would like couples to learn about child spacing. Then the children would be healthier and there would be enough food and jobs for everyone.

Putting contraceptives into milk to make people infertile is not possible. Nor would governments put contraceptives into other drinks or food.

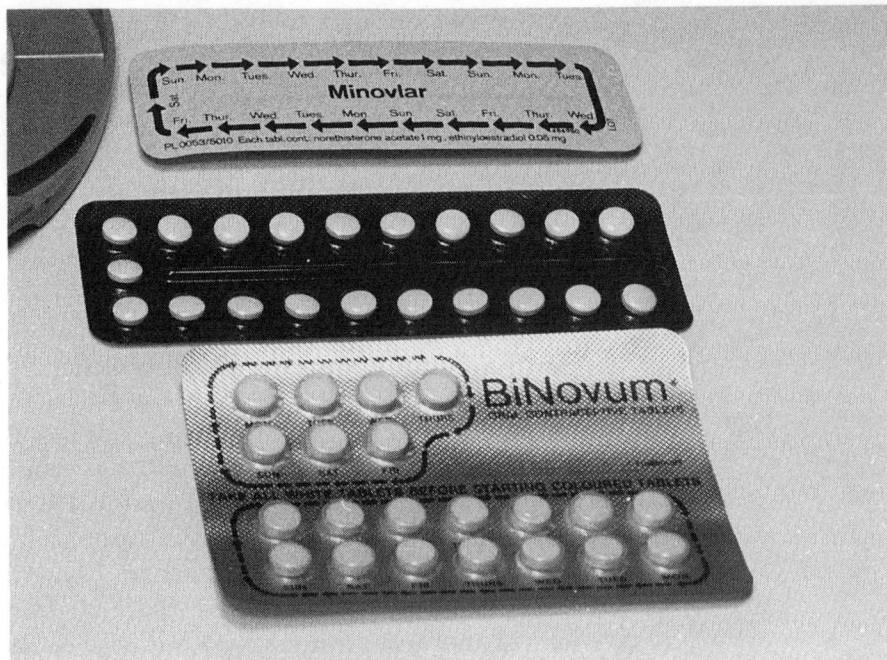

The Pill.

The Pill

What is the Pill?

The Pill is a tablet swallowed every day by the woman. The Pill comes in plastic packets containing one month's supply. Each day is marked to help the woman remember to take them. The Pill is a very reliable contraceptive if taken properly.

Every woman needs a health check-up before taking the Pill. She must tell the clinic about any diseases in her family and any medicines she is using. She should have her blood pressure measured and a health check-up by a health worker every six months, especially if she is having problems. In some countries the Pill can be bought from shops or markets. These Pills may be out-of-date or the shopkeeper may not understand the dangers of selling the Pill to any woman. Some pharmacists have been trained to sell the Pill.

Always get the Pill from a clinic or trained health worker.

How does the Pill work?

There are two types of contraceptive pill – the **Combined Pill** and the **Mini-Pill**. The Pill contains hormones which cause changes in the woman's body, similar to pregnancy. One of these changes is to stop ovulation. The woman has periods when she takes the Pill, but they are usually lighter and shorter. Both types of the Pill

80

prevent pregnancy but they have different effects on the woman's body. The Combined Pill is the most reliable but the Mini-Pill is safer for some women.

The Combined Pill contains two different hormones so it is more reliable in preventing pregnancy, but has more side effects than the Mini-Pill. The Combined Pill is not good for the health of some women.

Women who should **not** take the Combined Pill:
- Women smoking more than 15 cigarettes a day, if over 20 years old. (See Chapter 7, page 154.)
- Light smokers over 35 years old. They should give up first.
- Women over 45 years old.
- Breastfeeding mothers − because the milk production may be reduced. The Mini-Pill is safe.
- Women with severe **diabetes**.
- Women with heart or blood problems.
- Women with high blood pressure.
- Women with a past history of blood clots in the legs (not in menstrual flow).
- Women who are *very* overweight.
- Women with current **liver** or kidney diseases.
- *Severely* depressed women.
- Women confined to bed for a long time.
- Women having a *major* operation.
- Women with **sickle cell anaemia**

The Mini-Pill contains a smaller amount of one hormone. This hormone causes thick mucus in the cervix, so that sperm cannot travel through. Ovulation may occur, but the lining of the uterus does not prepare itself each month for a possible pregnancy.

The Mini-Pill has less side effects, but is not as reliable as the Combined Pill. Certain women should only take the Mini-Pill. The Mini-Pill is especially suitable for women over 30 years old. The woman swallows the Mini-Pill *every day of the month*, even during a period. The Mini-Pill *must* be taken at exactly the same time every day. If the Mini-Pill is taken more than three hours late, then the woman may become pregnant. She should take the pill but use additional contraception, such as a condom, for the next 14 days.

The Mini-Pill is safe for breastfeeding mothers. The Mini-Pill can be taken a week after childbirth.

A non-smoking woman with normal or low blood pressure could take the Mini-Pill until she is 50 years old.

There are many different brands and types of the Pill. Some are stronger than others. Every woman is different and needs a type of pill to suit her.

How is the Pill used?   The woman swallows one pill every day for 21 days. Then she stops for seven days while she has a period. She starts the next packet of pills after seven days even if she has had no period, or she is still bleeding. She is safe from pregnancy even during the seven days when she stops taking the Pill.

Some brands of the Pill have 28 pills in a packet. These are taken every day without stopping. Some women find it easier to remember to take a pill every day.

The Pill is started on the first day of the next period. The woman is safe from pregnancy at once. The next period will happen in about 23 days, but after that the periods will be every 28 days.

Most pregnancies on the Pill are caused by women forgetting to take the Pill every day. If a woman takes her pill a few hours late she should take the next one at the usual time.

If a woman forgets more than one pill, she should not take all the forgotten ones — she will probably vomit. She should take the next one and use a condom for 14 days, even if that means going on to the start of the next packet.

If she misses the next period she should visit the clinic to see if she is pregnant. The risk of pregnancy is higher if the forgotten pill was at the beginning of the packet. Forgetting the Mini-Pill carries more risk than forgetting the Combined Pill.

Take the Pill every day at the same time, not only after sex.

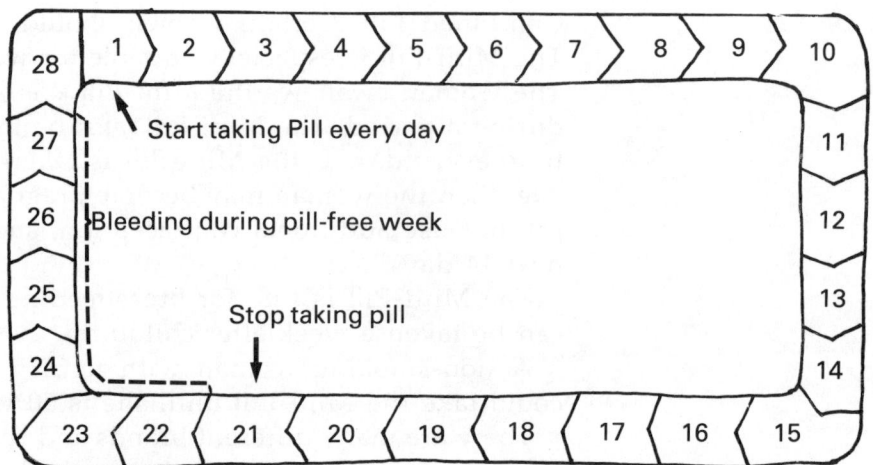

How to use the Pill.

If a woman has **diarrhoea or vomiting**, the Pill may not work. The Pill may be lost before it is absorbed into the body. If she vomited only once and more than three hours after taking the Pill, she is probably safe. Otherwise she should take another pill. If no more vomiting occurs, she is probably safe. If vomiting continues then she should take the Pill as usual but use a condom during intercourse for 14 days.

If severe diarrhoea continues for more than 24 hours, then take the pills as normal, but use a condom or diaphragm during intercourse for 14 days. Keep taking the pills whatever happens.

Taking just one pill will not prevent pregnancy.

There is no firm evidence of harm occurring to the baby if a woman gets pregnant while on the Pill.

When a woman wants to be pregnant she stops taking the Pill at the end of a packet. Her periods may take two or three months to return to normal. Her fertility will not be affected.

Starting the Pill after pregnancy

After pregnancy a woman can get pregnant before her first period. If breastfeeding, take the Mini-Pill four weeks after the birth. The Mini-Pill prevents pregnancy in a breastfeeding woman as effectively as the Combined Pill. The Combined Pill can be taken four weeks after birth if the baby is bottle fed. After a miscarriage or abortion start taking the Pill the next day. If there is any heavy bleeding in the first few weeks after a miscarriage, go to the clinic *quickly*.

If a child eats a packet of the Pill, there will not be any harmful results. The child may vomit or have nausea. One week later a girl child may have some painless bleeding from the vagina, like a light period. This will not affect her puberty.

Keep all medicines safely away from children.

Always keep a spare packet of the Pill with you. Many clinics give women six months' supply at a time. Make sure you return to the clinic *before* the last packet is finished.

Never take other medicines or drugs without telling the clinic that you are also taking the Pill. Certain medicines and drugs can stop each other working properly. Treatments for tuberculosis and epilepsy can interfere with the Pill. Other drugs may be affected by taking the Pill. Always tell the clinic of all drugs and medicines that you are taking. They may recommend that you change to another form of contraception.

Stop taking the Pill before a major operation. For minor operations such as female sterilization it is quite safe to continue taking the Pill.

| Always tell your doctor if you are taking the Pill. |

Is the Pill safe for a woman's health?

Every medicine has some **side-effects** and this includes the Pill. But taking the Pill is safer than having an unwanted pregnancy. For every 200 women who die in childbirth, only one woman will die from taking the Pill. The Pill makes periods easier for most women, but a few may suffer from unwanted side-effects.

Some of these are like the signs of early pregnancy. Sometimes changing the brand of the Pill helps. Most women have no side-effects while using the Pill. Many of the side-effects go away after two or three months of pill taking. The side-effects are:
- Headaches.
- Nausea in first few days of each packet. Usually goes away after two months. Take the Pill before going to sleep.
- Depression — eating liver, fish, milk, bananas and peanuts can help.
- Less desire for sex.
- Weight gain (see Chapter 7, page 148 for diets). Maximum weight is usually reached by the second month on the Pill.
- Light bleeding or 'spotting' between periods. Changing to a different type of the Pill may help.
- Inflamed gums — brush teeth regularly with a soft toothbrush or stick.
- Missed periods — this is not always a sign of pregnancy. Start taking the Pill again after seven days anyway. If two periods are missed then visit the clinic.
- Breast size increases.

Possibly dangerous side-effects — report these to the clinic quickly. Stop taking the Pill, but remember to use another contraceptive, such as a condom.
- Severe headaches.
- Sudden blurred eyesight.
- Flashing lights before the eyes.
- Severe leg, chest or abdominal pains.
- Heavy bleeding.
- Breathlessness after walking.
- Sudden weakness or tingling of hands or feet.
- Swelling of the legs.
- Fainting.
- Jaundice — yellow eyes.

> For most women the Pill is safer than unwanted pregnancy.

A woman can continue taking the Pill until she wants to get pregnant. She does not have to stop taking the Pill every two years.

Advantages of the Pill

- It is the most reliable contraceptive apart from sterilization. Out of 100 women taking the Combined Pill for a year less than one will get pregnant. Out of 100 women taking the Mini-Pill for a year three may get pregnant.
- It is easy to use.
- It does not interfere with lovemaking.
- It improves lovemaking by removing the worry of unwanted pregnancy.
- Pre-menstrual tension or depression may be reduced.
- Periods are lighter and shorter.
- Periods are regular: every 28 days.
- Period pains are less common.
- It relieves heavy periods and reduces the risk of anaemia.
- Pelvic infection is less common among women who take the Pill.
- It relieves acne and makes the skin less oily.
- It is easily reversible. When a woman wants to be pregnant, she simply stops taking the Pill. Her fertility will not be affected.
- Breast disease is less common.

Disadvantages of the Pill

- The Pill must be remembered *every* day. It is no good for forgetful women.
- The Pill affects the whole body and may have side-effects.
- Some women should not take the Pill.
- Women taking the Pill must visit the clinic for regular check-ups.
- Women over 35 years should *not* take the Combined Pill.
- Some women have a dry vagina and need extra lubrication during intercourse.
- If a couple only has sex once a month or less often, the woman must still take the Pill every day.

> There are no pills for men.

Dear Auntie,

My wife is taking contraceptive pills. What is surprising is that she unexpectedly enters into her menstrual periods. Is this normal?

Francis

Dear Francis,

A woman's periods on the Pill are usually much shorter with less blood because it is not a 'true' period. The uterus has not prepared itself for a fertilized egg, so the lining of the uterus is very thin. If your wife is bleeding between periods, then this is **breakthrough bleeding**. She may need a stronger type of Pill. If your wife takes the Pill every day, at the same time of day, then she should not become pregnant.

It does not matter if a woman has no periods while taking the Pill. Her normal periods will return when she stops taking the Pill and she will get pregnant as easily as before.

Every woman on the Pill should have a regular health check-up at the child spacing clinic. The health workers there will answer any questions or worries.

Dear Auntie,

Is it true that the Pill makes women get cancer?

Suzie

Dear Suzie,

Studies have been done in different parts of the world to find out if there is any connection between cancer and the Pill. There may be a small connection between the Pill and some types of cancer, though this has not been proved. What is certain is that cancer of the ovary and of the lining of the womb occur less often among women taking the Pill than other women.

In a healthy woman, risk from unwanted pregnancy is always greater than the health risk from taking the Pill.

Injectable contraceptive, or the shot

What is the shot?

An Injectable, or the shot is an injection of hormones given to a woman every two or three months, depending on the brand. It is also called Depo, Depo-Provera, or Norigest (brand names).

How does the shot work?

An injection in the woman's arm or bottom slowly releases hormones in the body similar to the hormones in the Mini-Pill. These hormones stop ovulation and make extra thick mucus in the cervix which prevents sperm reaching the uterus.

How is the shot used?

Every two or three months the woman visits the clinic for an injection. The couples must use another contraceptive, such as a condom, for two weeks after the first injection.

Advantages of the shot

• There is nothing to remember except for one visit to the clinic every two or three months.
• If the woman forgets to go to the clinic, she should be safe for a few days.
• No-one knows the woman is using the shot.
• Nothing interferes with lovemaking.
• The shot is a very reliable contraceptive. Out of 400 women using it in one year only *one* will get pregnant.
• Some women prefer one injection every two or three months to taking pills every day.
• The shot is safe for breastfeeding mothers and helps make more milk. The shot is best given to a mother four weeks after childbirth.
• Many woman have no periods after a year of using the shot. This does no harm and some women like this.
   The shot is safe for women:
— With sickle-cell disease. The shot helps this.
— Who smoke cigarettes.
— Who forget to use other methods.
— Who find other methods difficult.
— Who have had all the children they want.
— Who are over 35 years.

Disadvantages of the shot

• Irregular periods are common. Most women have no periods after a year of using the shot. They may worry that they have become pregnant or infertile.
• Side-effects can include headaches, dizziness, depression, bleeding between periods or heavy periods. Any of these should be reported to the clinic immediately.
• If there are side-effects, the woman has to wait until the shot stops working. She cannot stop the shot immediately.

● If a woman wants to have a baby, it may take 6 to 12 months before her periods are normal and she is fertile again. Once her periods have started, her fertility will be as good as before.

Women who should not usually use the shot:

— Young women.
— Women with no children.
— Women with diabetes.
— Women with heavy periods.
— Women with very irregular periods.

Women should always have the shot carefully explained to them. In some places women are given the shot without understanding its effects and how it works.

Intra-Uterine Device, or IUD

What is an IUD?   'Intra-uterine' means 'inside the **uterus** or womb'. A device is an object or thing. An IUD is a piece of plastic about 2 cm long that is placed inside the uterus of a woman. Some IUDs are made of plastic, coated with copper metal. Some copper IUDs are changed every three years, though some can be safely left inside the uterus for many years. Other names for IUD are coil, loop, T device, Copper 7 and IUCD — intra-uterine contraceptive device.

How does the IUD work?   The IUD prevents a fertilized ovum from staying in the uterus. The woman has periods in the normal way, but they may be heavier for the first few months as the uterus gets used to the IUD.

How is the IUD used?   The IUD is inserted into the uterus through the vagina at a clinic. The woman lies on her back and the nurse or doctor carefully inserts the IUD using a long thin tube. The tube is removed from the vagina and the IUD stays in the uterus. The woman may feel pain for a few seconds. Many women feel nothing. The IUD has a string on the end so the woman can feel it is there.

Some clinics prefer to insert the IUD during or just after a menstrual period. Then they know that the woman is not already pregnant. The IUD can be fitted four to six weeks after birth, before the woman starts menstruating again.

Advantages of the IUD   ● The IUD prevents pregnancy from the day it is fitted. The woman can then forget about contraception.
● The husband cannot feel the IUD.
● When the woman wants a baby the IUD is easily removed at a

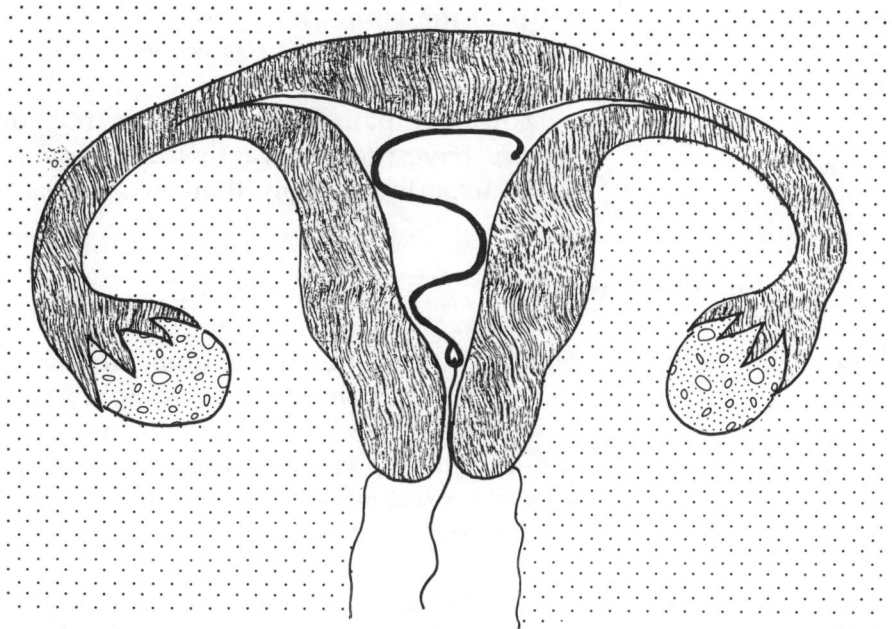

Inserting an IUD into the uterus

clinic. The best time is during a period. IUDs should never be removed by the user at home — this could damage the uterus. The woman is immediately fertile again.

● The woman only has to visit a clinic once a year.

● The IUD can be used as a **post-coital** contraceptive. (See page 112.)

● For every 100 women using an IUD for a year, three will become pregnant.

Disadvantages of the IUD

● For the first few months periods can be heavier and longer than normal.

● Some women have strong period pains. Women with normally heavy or long periods should not use the IUD.

● Infections of the uterus are more common with an IUD, especially if the woman or man has several partners. Infections can make a woman infertile. Any signs of fever, pain or discharge should be reported to the clinic.

● The IUD can occasionally fall out. The woman must feel for the string after each period. If she cannot feel it she must return to the clinic. Meanwhile, she should use another contraceptive, such as the condom.

● Pregnancy with an IUD can occur in the fallopian tube. This is rare, but dangerous. An operation is necessary to prevent major bleeding.

Go to the clinic if:

— You think the IUD has come out because you cannot feel the threads.

— You have pain especially with intercourse.

— You have unusual vaginal discharge.

— Your period is more than two weeks late.

The cap, or diaphragm

What is the cap?

The cap is a round cup or dome about 6 cm across made of thin rubber. Other names include diaphragm and dutch cap. The cap is kept in shape with a springy metal rim which is encased in rubber. The cap is made from thicker rubber than the condom, so it can be used many times. Caps usually last for one or two years if properly cared for.

How does the cap work?

Every time a couple have intercourse the cap is placed over the cervix, in the woman's vagina beforehand. This stops the sperm entering the uterus and reaching the ovum. The cap is left inside the woman for six hours after intercourse. The cap cannot get lost inside the woman. It is held in place by the muscles of the vagina. It cannot fall out and it does not get in the way of intercourse.

The cap should be used with **spermicide**. The spermicide forms

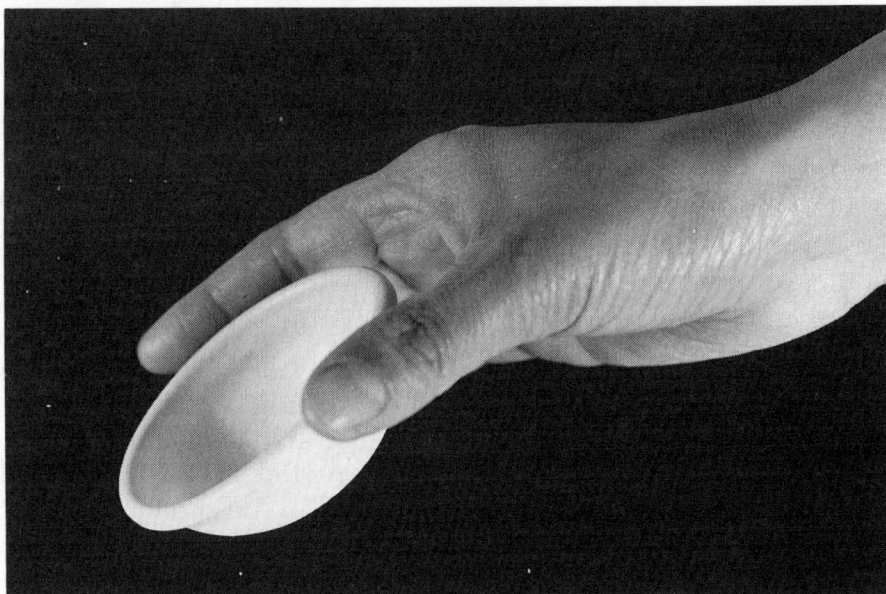

The cap.

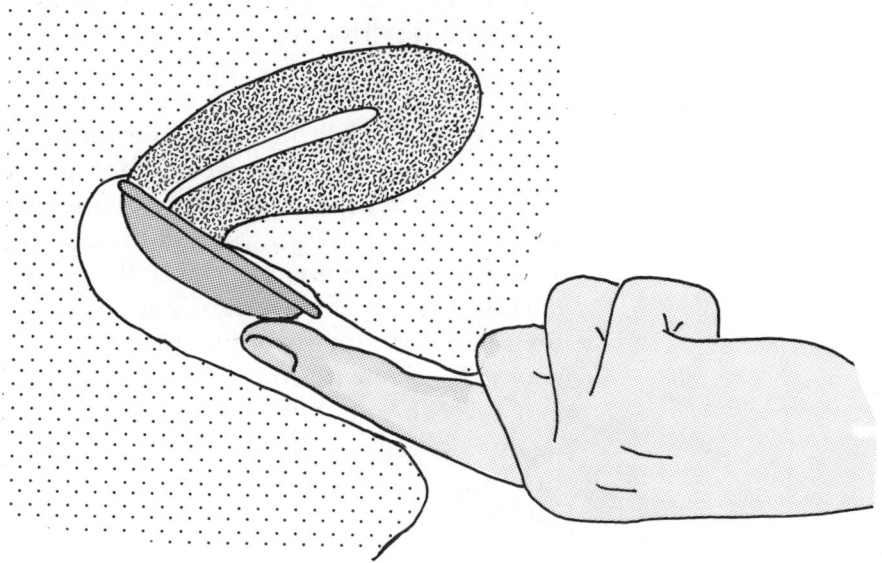

Putting in a cap

a seal and kills any sperm swimming near the cap.

Every woman is a slightly different size inside, so there are different sizes of caps. The cap is fitted at a clinic to get the correct size for each woman. After having a baby, or putting on a lot of weight, a woman's vagina may have grown. She must visit her clinic to check the cap still fits.

How is the cap used?

The clinic will show the woman how to insert the cap and spermicide. She should practise at home before she needs it for intercourse. If she uses it in a hurry without practice, she may not put it in correctly.

Wash the hands. Squeeze two strips of spermicide on both sides of the cap. Bend the cap edge flat between the fingers and thumb and push it up into the vagina so that the cervix is covered. Always check that the cap is correctly in place by feeling with the middle finger. If the cap is not covering the cervix, then take it out and start again.

Some women put the cap in every night, in case they want to make love. This is the best way. Other women wait until love-making starts, and then stop to put it in. With practice putting the cap in only takes a few seconds.

If the cap is inserted more than three hours before intercourse then more spermicide should be put in the vagina. The cap must be left inside for at least six hours after intercourse. The cap can be left in for up to 24 hours.

The cap should also be used for intercourse during a menstrual period. If a period starts while the cap is inside, just remove it as usual after intercourse.

After removing the cap, wash it gently in mild soap and warm water. Rinse it with clean water and dry it carefully with a clean towel. Never put the cap in hot or boiling water. Never use detergents, washing powder, disinfectants, strong soap, talcum powder, vegetable oil, petroleum jelly or face cream with the cap. These will rot the rubber and stop the spermicide working.

Hold the cap up to the light to check for any holes or cracks. Sperm can swim through even a very small hole. Keep it in a cool, dry, clean place.

If the cap gets out of shape the rim can be gently bent round again. Go back to the clinic every six months to check the cap still fits. Never use a friend's cap — she may not be the same size inside.

Advantages of the cap

- There are no health risks.
- There is no effect on a woman's periods.
- Women of all ages can use the cap.
- It is only used when intercourse occurs. This makes it suitable

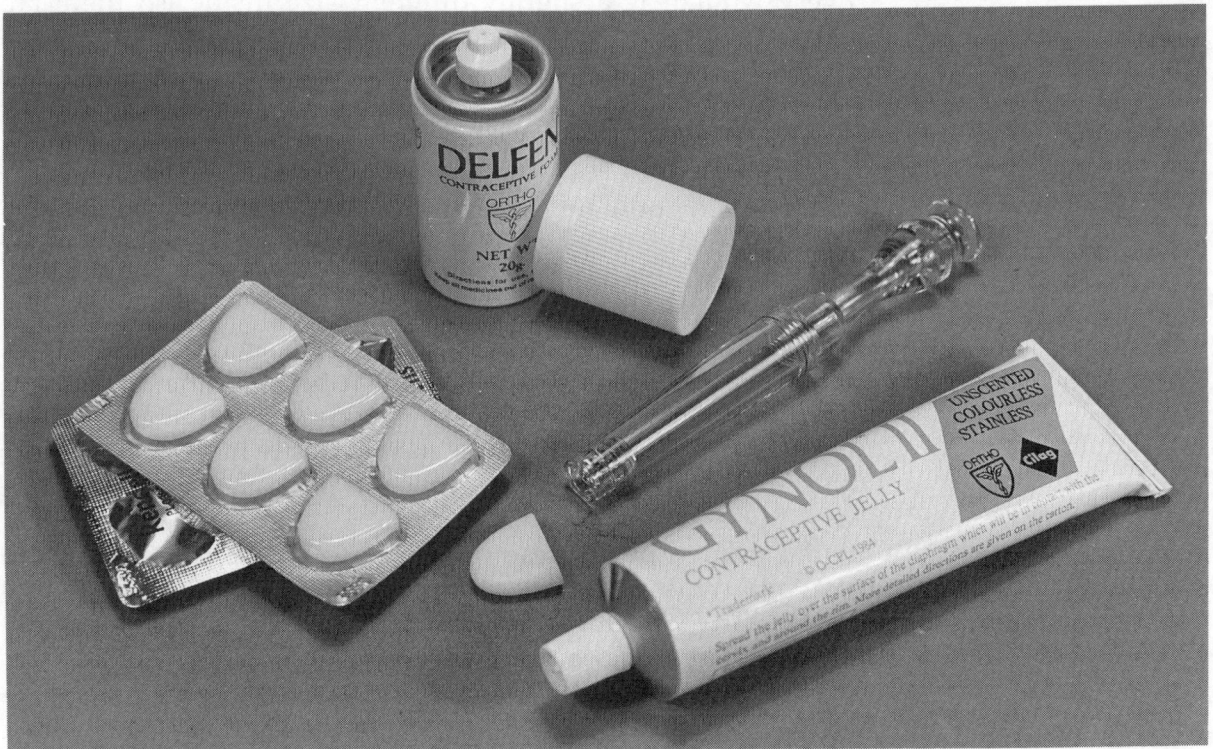

Spermicides.

for woman who have intercourse rarely. For example, if their husbands work away from home.
- It is cheap, and available in most clinics.
- The woman cannot feel the cap inside her.
- If the couple do not like the cap, they can easily change to another method of contraception.
- For every 100 women using the cap correctly for a year, only three women will get pregnant.

Disadvantages of the cap

- The cap and spermicide must be used *every* time and *never* forgotten. The woman must remember to take the cap and spermicide around with her.
- Some women do not like putting the cap inside the vagina.
- Some couples find the spermicide messy. They may be using too much.
- In a home with no bathroom, the cap can be embarrassing for a woman to use.
- If there is no running water, there is a danger of infection if the cap is not kept very clean.
- The penis may occasionally push the cap out of place. This is why spermicide must be used with the cap.

Spermicide

What is spermicide?

Spermicide is a chemical which destroys sperm in the vagina to prevent pregnancy. It is a cream, jelly or foam.

How does spermicide work?

Spermicide destroys the sperm when they reach the vagina, during sexual intercourse. Spermicide does not harm the woman — only the sperm. Spermicide should be used with another method of contraception such as the condom or the cap.

How is spermicide used?

Spermicide creams are most suitable for use with caps and condoms. The woman puts the spermicide cream on the cap before inserting it, to prevent any sperm swimming underneath the cap and into the uterus. (See page 91 on how to use the cap.)

When using a condom a man can put spermicide on his penis and on the condom in case he should withdraw too late after intercourse. The spermicide will destroy any sperm that spill out.

Spermicide can also be bought in **pessaries**. These are solid jelly tablets that look like sweets. One pessary is placed in the vagina and pushed as far inside as possible with the finger or with a plastic applicator. The spermicide works after about 10 to 15 minutes, when the warmth of the body makes the jelly melt.

Foam spermicide comes in an aerosol tin. The foam is squirted from the tin into a plastic applicator. The applicator places the correct amount of foam in the vagina. The applicator is then removed.

Advantages of spermicide

- There is no known risk to a woman's health.
- It can be bought in most pharmacies as well as clinics.
- Spermicide used correctly with a cap or condom is a reliable contraceptive. For every 100 women using this method for a year, only three will get pregnant.
- It can help make intercourse more comfortable by lubricating the vagina.
- It reduces the risk of pregnancy if sperm spills.

Disadvantages of spermicide

- Spermicides can be messy.
- Spermicides are not poisonous, but some men do not like the taste of spermicide during **oral sex**.
- Pessary spermicides take up to 15 minutes to melt and become effective.
- After three hours most spermicides stop working and must be re-applied.
- Spermicide should not be used without a cap.
- Occasionally the sensitive skin of the vagina may be irritated by the spermicides.
- The couple must keep the spermicide near their bed for when they make love.
- Spermicide must be used *every* time a couple make love.
- Spermicides do not work if inserted *after* intercourse.

Spermicides should be used with a condom or a cap.

Douche

What is a douche?

A douche is a plastic bag rather like a toy balloon with a long narrow end. The bag is filled with soap and warm water, or spermicide and water. Immediately after a couple have finished making love the woman squirts the water inside her vagina. Another similar method that is often tried is squirting fizzy cool drinks up the vagina.

How does the douche work?

Douching is meant to wash out all the sperm after intercourse. But sperm move fast and many of them will already be in the uterus when the douche is used, even if it is only a few minutes after intercourse. The liquid can push more sperm into the uterus.

Disadvantages of the douche	• The douche is a poor contraceptive with a very high failure rate.
	• The spermicide or soap can cause vaginal irritation or soreness.
	• The vagina can become infected if the water or douche bag are not very clean.
	• The couple have to think about contraception very fast after making love. The douche has to be used within seconds of intercourse. This can ruin relaxed lovemaking.
	• Vaginal douching is messy. The woman has to crouch in a bath or over a toilet as the liquid runs out of her vagina.
	• Douching should never be considered as a contraceptive.
	• This is *not* a reliable contraceptive and may encourage pregnancy by pushing the sperm into the uterus. Sperm may swim into the uterus in less than two minutes.

The natural method

What is the natural method?	The natural method of contraception helps a woman to understand when she is going to ovulate and when she might therefore get pregnant if she has intercourse. The couple stop having intercourse during the **fertile days** when the woman could get pregnant.
	This method also works for couples planning a pregnancy. They have intercourse only on the fertile days.
How does it work?	As described in Chapter 2, page 21, an ovum is made inside the woman every month about 14 days before a period. Certain signs show a woman the fertile days when intercourse can lead to pregnancy. The ovum lives for up to 24 hours and a man's sperm can live for seven days inside the woman. The fertile time is about eight days in each month, or menstrual cycle.
	A woman can find the fertile time if she observes her body temperature, her vaginal mucus, her cervix and the dates of her periods. When a woman has learnt how to observe all these changes in her body then she can estimate the fertile days when she could become pregnant. Young women should learn how to do this long before they get married. Six months may be needed to work out a woman's menstrual cycle and pattern of ovulation.
	1 Periods, or the rhythm method
	Every month the woman marks on a calendar the days of her period. After a few months she will notice a pattern − her periods come at regular intervals that may vary by a few days each month. Some women have 'short cycles' of about 20 days

Shortest known cycle **26** days
Length of this cycle **28** days

Route of temperature | O ✓ | V | R
Time of taking temperature **8 a.m.**

Name **MARY**

Number **2**

Month **JUNE**

KEY

P	Period or blood loss
D	Dry day
M	Mucus
F	Fertile–type mucus
✗	Peak day
—	Beginning of probably fertile days
1 2 3	Days after Peak Day

Body temperature (37.5 down to 35.5)

Sexual Intercourse
Days of the Menstrual Cycle: 1 2 3 4 5 6 7 8 9 10 11 12 13 14 15 16 17 18 19 20 21 22 23 24 25 26 27 28 29 30 31 32 33 34 35 36 37 38 39 40

P P P P P D D M M M F ✗ 1 2 3 4 5 ... P

Mucus–Sensation / Appearance / Stretch: No mucus, no mucus, no mucus, wet, thin mucus, slippery, slippery, sticky, sticky, dry

Cyclical Symptoms: Tender breasts

Cervix–Rising / Opening / Softening / Tilt: ✗ ✗ ✗

Temperature and mucus chart.

and other women have 'long cycles' of up to 35 days. Most women cannot get pregnant during the 10 days before a period. Women with short cycles can get pregnant during a period or in the days after a period. The idea of the rhythm method is to calculate the fertile days. The woman may get pregnant if she has intercourse during this time. Illness or worry can change the pattern of a woman's periods and make them irregular. This makes it difficult to calculate the fertile days exactly.

2 Body temperature

The woman needs a special **thermometer**, which shows the very small changes in a woman's body temperature during each menstrual cycle. The normal body temperature is 37°C. When ovulation occurs, the body temperature rises very slightly — by about half a degree Centigrade. An ordinary clinical thermometer does not show this small rise so well.

Every morning the woman puts the thermometer in her mouth or in her vagina for five minutes before she gets out of bed or drinks anything. She marks her temperature on a special chart. After doing this every day for a month or two she will notice that about 14 days before her next period her temperature rises for a few days. This small rise in temperature shows that ovulation is happening. The temperature goes down again just before the next period. Fevers, illness or worry can upset a woman's body temperature, but these temperature changes will be larger than the small rises at ovulation. Some medicines such as aspirin can change the normal body temperature.

After a few months a woman can tell exactly when ovulation has occurred and know when intercourse is safer. The woman can only know when she has ovulated. She cannot tell before she ovulates exactly when it will occur. If a couple have intercourse a day or two *before* ovulation, then the sperm could stay alive and wait to fertilize the ovum.

After the temperature has risen for three days the couple can have intercourse with a low risk of pregnancy.

3   Mucus

Every day, except during her period, the woman has to observe the **mucus** in her vagina. She can do this with a clean finger or a piece of toilet paper. During most of the cycle the mucus is sticky like paste. It is cloudy white and does not stretch.

During the fertile days the mucus is slippery and clear, like raw egg white. This fertile mucus stretches for 3 or 4 cm between the fingers. The fertile mucus usually occurs for a few days half way between two periods at the time of ovulation. The vagina feels wet. Slippery fertile mucus helps the sperm to travel up the vagina and uterus to the ovum. When the mucus is clear and slippery then ovulation is happening. The woman will probably get pregnant if she has intercourse during or before this time without using a contraceptive.

The woman should note the type of mucus and wetness every day on her calendar or chart. She needs no special equipment to do this. When she has had four days with no slippery mucus she is safe. Intercourse should stop as soon as the mucus is noticed and for four days after the fertile mucus has finished.

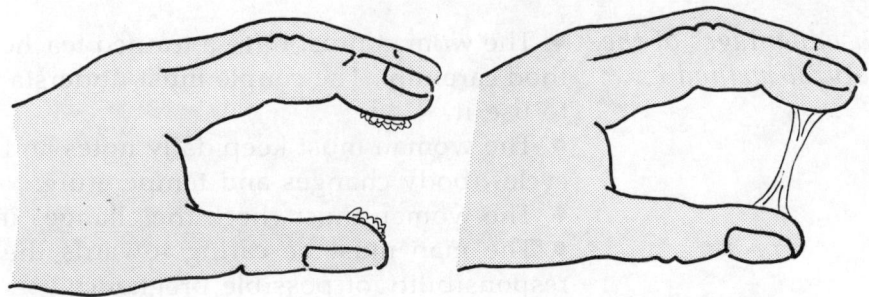

Changes in mucus.

Women with a short cycle will notice the slippery fertile mucus soon after the end of their periods. Women with a cycle of about 28 days will notice the slippery fertile mucus about 10 days after their period ends.

4 Cervix

After a period the cervix is low in the vagina. A woman can easily reach it with her fingers. It feels hard, like the top of a nose. During the fertile days the cervix rises higher into the vagina and is more difficult to reach. It feels soft with a hole in the middle, like pouting lips. After ovulation, when the fertile days are finished the cervix drops lower and becomes hard again.

By combining all these signs of the fertile days, a woman can work out on which days intercourse is safe.

When a couple want to have a baby they can have sexual intercourse during the fertile days to increase the possibility of pregnancy.

Advantages of natural methods

- There are no harmful effects on health, except unwanted pregnancy.
- It is good for couples with a lasting relationship. Shared responsibility is the key to this method.
- Co-operation between the partners can increase their love and understanding.
- It encourages couples to explore other ways of lovemaking apart from intercourse.
- Some couples enjoy intercourse more after a time of abstinence.
- Women become aware of their body's changes and fertility. Men learn about their wives' bodies.
- Teachers of this method do not have to be qualified doctors or nurses. They can be school teachers or village health workers.
- There are no contraceptive devices, such as condoms, to interfere with intercourse.
- It helps women get pregnant when they want to.
- The success rate is high if the couples understand the method and use it properly.
- It is approved by the Catholic Church.

Disadvantages of the natural method

- The woman must have a trained teacher who explains this method carefully. The couple must understand the method and how to use it.
- The woman must keep daily notes and charts of her menstrual cycles, body changes and temperature.
- The woman must check the changes in her body every day.
- The man must be caring towards the woman and share the responsibility of possible pregnancy.
- It needs a strong will and co-operation between both partners.

During the fertile days the couple cannot have sexual intercourse, or any contact between the penis and vagina.

• This is not a method for couples who rarely see each other. If the man works away from home and only visits his wife occasionally, he will not be pleased if she says, 'I'm sorry, we cannot make love this week'.

• Some women feel nervous making love because they worry about the possibility of pregnancy.

• Every woman has a different menstrual cycle and pattern of fertile days.

• It is more difficult for women with irregular periods.

• Sperm may live for over a week in the uterus, waiting for an ovum.

• It is more difficult for women after childbirth, during breast-feeding or for older women approaching the menopause.

• For every 100 couples who really understand and use the natural method about five women will get pregnant. For most couples using this method about 25 women in 100 will get pregnant.

Condom

What is the condom? The **condom** is a tube of smooth rubber worn over the man's penis during intercourse. The rubber is very thin and stretchy so it fits tightly over all sizes of erect penis. Most condoms are a pale colour. Red, green, pink, blue and black condoms are also sold. Some condoms are ribbed or have bumps around the end. This can give the woman extra pleasure but has no extra effect in preventing pregnancy. The condom is also called the **sheath,** protective, **Durex**, (brand name), rubber, french letter or rubber johnny.

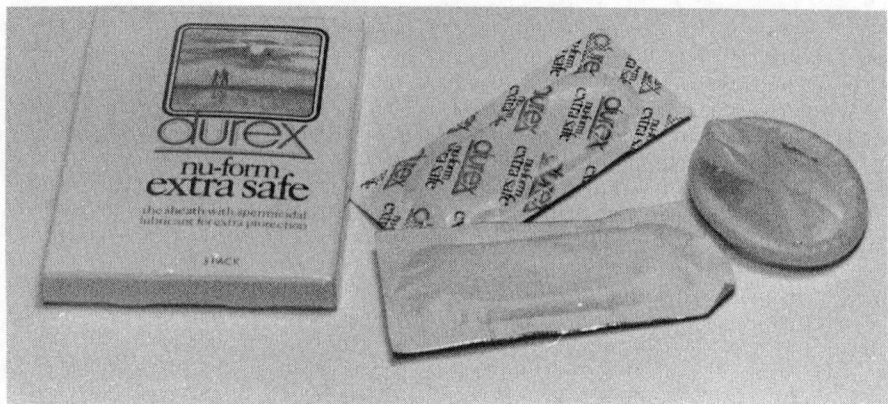

Condoms.

| How does the condom work? | The condom catches the semen at ejaculation and prevents the sperm swimming up inside the woman's vagina. Most condoms have a narrow tip, like a nipple to catch the semen. The condom is one of the oldest and most popular methods of contraception. It is the only reliable method available to men, except for sterilization. |

How does the condom work?

The condom catches the semen at ejaculation and prevents the sperm swimming up inside the woman's vagina. Most condoms have a narrow tip, like a nipple to catch the semen. The condom is one of the oldest and most popular methods of contraception. It is the only reliable method available to men, except for sterilization.

How is the condom used?

The condom is put on the erect penis before there is any contact between the penis and the vagina. Drops of semen often come out of the penis before ejaculation. One drop of semen can contain 3 or 4 million sperm. The condom will not stay on if it is put on before an erection — the erection will push it off.

When the condom is bought it may be wrapped in foil to protect it from dirt and damage. The condom is rolled into a small circle.

Do not unroll the sheath before putting it on. The rolled up condom is placed over the glans (head) of the penis as soon as it is hard. Squeeze the closed end of the condom between the fingers to push out the air. The end or the nipple of the condom

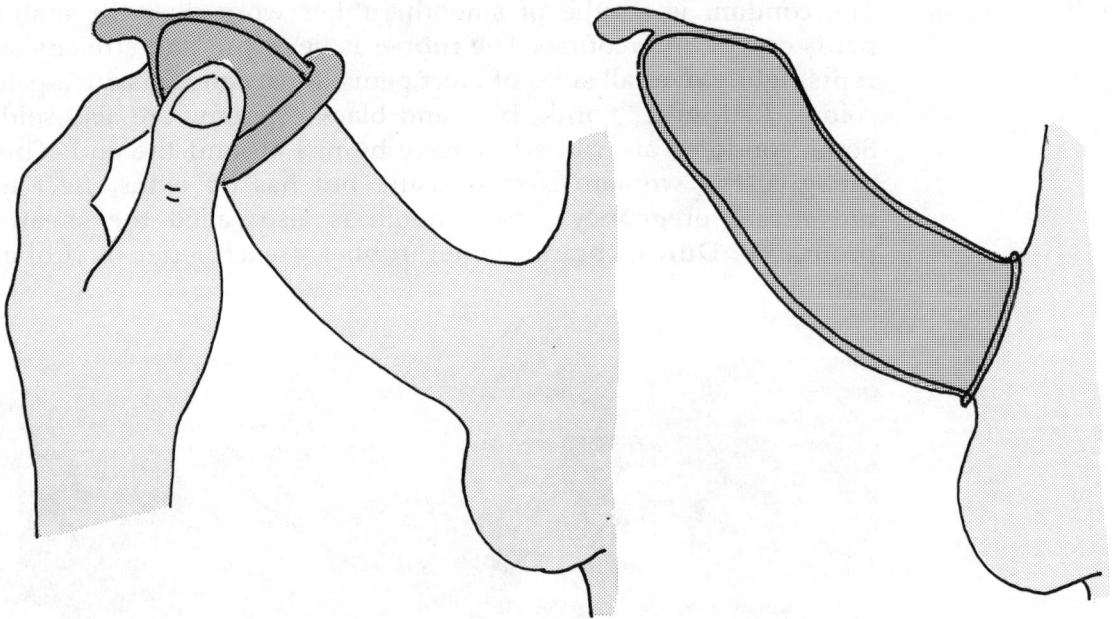

Putting on a condom.

100

must be left empty to catch the semen at ejaculation. Then gently unroll the condom evenly down the full length of the penis. Trying to pull it on like a sock may break it. With practice this can be done with one hand in a few seconds. Some women do this for their partner as part of their lovemaking. This way lovemaking is not interrupted and the man will not lose his erection. Beware of sharp nails or jewelled rings as these can tear the thin rubber.

If a man has never used a condom he can practise putting one on when he is alone. This may save time and embarrassment later with his partner.

The man can hardly feel the condom when it is on and many women cannot feel it during intercourse. Most condoms are coated with a thin layer of oil to make intercourse more comfortable for both partners. Some condoms are coated with spermicide. If the sheath should fall off, then this gives extra protection against pregnancy.

After ejaculation the man should withdraw his penis slowly before it becomes soft, holding the sheath firmly so that no semen is spilt. If the penis remains inside after it has become soft then the condom may fall off inside the woman. This could lead to pregnancy.

Afterwards keep the penis away from the woman's body — it will be covered in live sperm. Wrap the used condom in paper and flush it down the toilet or put it in a dustbin.

Use a new condom *every* time you make love. If a couple cannot be bothered because the condom is in another room, or they have forgotten to buy some more, the woman may get pregnant. For extra protection use a condom together with spermicide jelly, cream, or foam (see page 93).

Keep a packet of condoms next to the bed, or in your pocket so that they are nearby when they are needed. If you have to go and look for the condoms in the middle of lovemaking, then you may find your partner has fallen asleep when you return!

Never keep condoms in a hot place or in sunlight. Never use a condom which is over a year old. If the date on the packet has passed, then the condom could tear. Never use petroleum jelly or face cream for lubrication with condoms. Petroleum jelly rots rubber and face cream irritates the sensitive skin of the vagina. Special lubrication jellies are available in shops and clinics. Water-based jellies such as 'KY' jelly can be used.

Never put two condoms on at once. Some couples think this will give them extra protection, but the condoms are more likely to tear by rubbing against each other.

Use a new condom each time you make love, even if you make love several times in one night. In emergencies a condom can be washed with soap and water and used again. This is not recommended because a washed condom can break or develop small holes. The saving made by re-using a condom is not worth the risk of an unwanted pregnancy. The cheapest condoms without a brand name are the least reliable and may tear in use. Durex is a reliable brand.

Condoms are usually sold in packets of three or twelve. If the shopkeeper asks 'What size?' he means 'How many condoms?' not 'How big is your penis?'! If you are shy about asking, then write it down on a piece of paper.

Warning: There is a type of condom sometimes called 'American Tips'. This covers only the end of the penis. These do not work. They fall off inside the vagina or the sperm leak out of the sides. Never use this type.

Advantages of the condom

- They are cheap and easy to buy. You can find them in pharmacies, barber's shops, clinics and bars.
- In some countries condoms are free or very cheap from clinics.
- They need no fitting or visits to the clinic.
- It is the only easy method of contraception available to men.
- When a man uses a condom it shows that he cares about his partner.
- They have no effect on the health of either the man or the woman. The condom does not interfere with the menstrual cycle or with the insides of either partner's body.
- Used *every* time, the condom is one of the most reliable methods of contraception. For every 100 couples using the condom correctly for a year, only two or three women will get pregnant.
- Condoms can help with lovemaking. Men who ejaculate quickly find that wearing a condom may delay ejaculation. This gives them and their partners longer pleasure.
- Condoms require no previous planning or fitting, except to have the condoms ready.
- Condoms work immediately and are seen to be used. This can give couples greater confidence and therefore help their love-making to be more relaxed.
- They are particularly suitable for men who have no permanent partner. These men can carry a packet of condoms with them and always be safe. No man should assume that his partner is using a contraceptive.
- A condom protects both partners against sexually transmitted diseases, such as gonorrhoea and AIDS. A condom cannot guarantee protection, but it may help.

Disadvantages of the condom

- A new condom must be used every time that a couple makes love.

- Putting the condom on can be an interruption for an inexperienced couple.
- Some couples do not like the rubber smell of condoms. The cheaper brands smell more than the better quality brands, like Durex.
- Some men find that the condom reduces the sensations felt by the penis. What a man loses in sensations, he gains in the length of time he can make love before ejaculating. This can be an advantage to men who ejaculate too soon, and more enjoyable for the woman.

Caring men always carry condoms.

Pulling Out or interrupted intercourse, coitus interruptus

What is Pulling Out?

The man takes his penis out of the vagina just before he ejaculates, or 'comes'. He then ejaculates outside the woman.

How does Pulling Out work?

The idea is that if the man ejaculates outside the woman, then none of the sperm will get inside the woman and fertilize the ovum.

Advantages of Pulling Out

- There is nothing to buy, so it is free.
- No planning is needed. Pulling out is always available.
- No clinic visits are needed.
- There are no health risks as no drugs or devices are used. The main health risk is an unwanted pregnancy.
- It is better than doing nothing at all.

Disadvantages of Pulling Out

- Before a man ejaculates fully, some of the sperm leaks out of his penis. So while the penis is inside the vagina, some of these sperm can cause pregnancy.
- Many men do not know exactly when they are going to ejaculate. They may pull their penises out too late.
- If the man ejaculates near the vagina some of the sperm can swim through the mucus of the vulva and up into the vagina.
- The man cannot fully enjoy his orgasm. He must concentrate on pulling out in time.
- The man may forget to pull out.
- The woman gets less satisfaction from this method as the penis may be pulled out before she has reached orgasm too.

103

● Both partners may worry so much about the risk of pregnancy that they cannot enjoy making love.
● For every 100 women using this method for a year about 20 will get pregnant.

Vasectomy

What is a vasectomy?

A **vasectomy** is a small operation performed on a man to make him unable to create babies. The sperm duct, or vas, in the scrotum is cut on each side and sewn apart.

How does a vasectomy work?

Many millions of sperm are made in the man's two testicles. The semen is made in glands near the bladder. After a vasectomy the sperm cannot travel from the testicles to the penis, so a man cannot make a woman pregnant. Semen is still made and is ejaculated through the penis at orgasm with the same feelings to the man.

If a couple have had all the children they want, the man can have a vasectomy. After discussing this with his doctor the man goes to the clinic or hospital. He washes his genitals and an **injection** is made near them so that he cannot feel anything. The doctor cuts a small hole 1 to 2 cm long in the skin of the scrotum, under the penis. The doctor cuts each of the two vas. He ties the

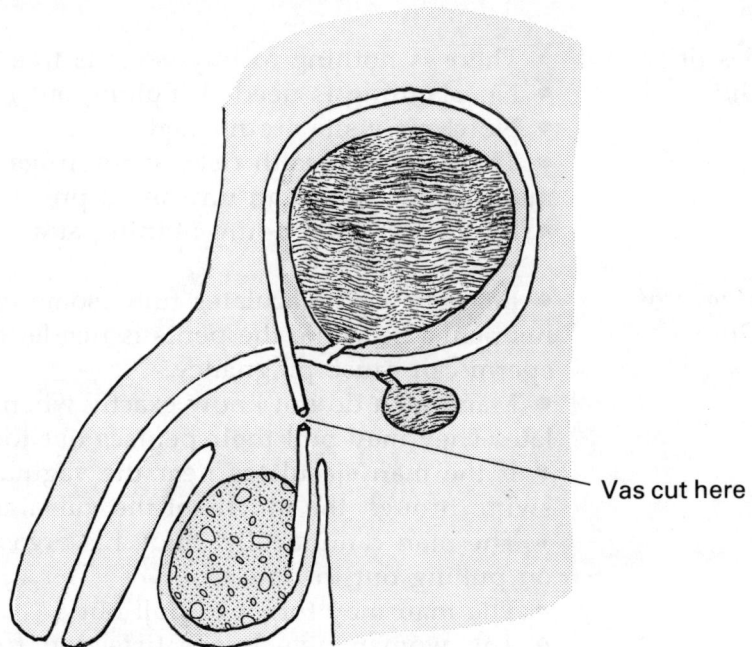

Vas cut here

Vasectomy.

ends to prevent them growing together again. The doctor sews up the cut with one or two stitches. The operation takes about ten minutes. After a short rest the man can return home. The injection wears off after about an hour and the testicles may feel sore for a day or two. Tight fitting pants will help support them. Aspirin or other painkilling tablets will ease the soreness. Alcohol is not good as it can increase bleeding.

The scrotum heals very quickly and the stitches fall out after a few days. The man should not wash the scrotum for 48 hours. He should avoid carrying heavy weights for a few days.

How is a vasectomy used?

The man can have intercourse as soon as he feels like it. But the couple must use another contraceptive, such as a condom, until there are no sperm in the semen.

For most men the sperm should be finished after about 12 ejaculations. At the hospital he ejaculates into a clean jar and the semen is examined for sperm. The sperm is tested again after a few weeks. If there are no sperm in the semen, then the man can have intercourse with no risk of pregnancy in his wife.

Sometimes the man is given 15 condoms, to be used each time he has intercourse. When these 15 condoms are finished, the couple is free to make love without using any protection.

In some countries vasectomy is the most widely used method of contraception by married couples who have had children.

Dear Auntie,

My wife and I have four beautiful children. After the birth of the youngest one my wife was very ill. The doctors said she must not take the Pill, but they also said that another pregnancy could kill her. My cousin had an operation to stop his wife becoming pregnant. But I am worried that if I had this operation I would not desire my wife any more. Would I become a woman?

Moses

Dear Moses,

The operation you speak of is a vasectomy, or cutting the sperm ducts. After a vasectomy a man still produces male hormones, as the testicles and penis are not removed. You will still desire your wife as strongly as before. During lovemaking you still have an erection, and semen comes out when you come. But your wife cannot ever get pregnant again. A vasectomy is the best present that a loving man can give to his wife.

Advantages of a vasectomy	• After a vasectomy a man has sexual intercourse in the same way as before. Neither he nor his wife will feel any difference. He still has erections and ejaculations. The only difference is that there are no sperm in the semen.
	• Many couples find making love is better after a vasectomy, because they no longer worry about contraception or unwanted pregnancy.
	• There are no interruptions during lovemaking and so a couple can just enjoy themselves.
	• Most couples have had all the children they want by the age of 35 years, but the man will be fertile for the rest of his life, perhaps for another 35 years.
	• Vasectomy is good for couples who are forgetful about contraception. They never have to remember it again.
	• The operation only takes a few minutes in an out-patient clinic or hospital.
	• A vasectomy is easier, quicker and safer than the sterilization operation for women.
	• In some countries the operation is free, or costs very little.
	• A vasectomy does not interfere with the woman's health or menstrual periods. It is a good method if a woman's life would be in danger if she became pregnant again.
	• Having a vasectomy is a way a man can show he really cares for his wife. He has taken responsibility for contraception.
	• There is no health risk to the man. After vasectomies, men continue to be sportsmen, film stars, labourers and teachers.
	• The testicles still make male sex hormones, so the man still grows a beard and is attracted to women. The man's virility and performance are not affected.
	• There are no scars after a vasectomy. The man may be able to feel two small lumps in his scrotum where the vas have been cut. Apart from his wife and doctor, no-one else will know unless he tells them.
	• Vasectomy is the most effective contraception available. For every 2000 couples using this method for a year, only one woman will get pregnant. There is a very rare chance that the vas grow together again.
Disadvantages of vasectomy	• It is not a method for young unmarried men.
	• The couple must be sure that they have got all the children they want.
	• In most cases vasectomy cannot be reversed. Some doctors ask the couple to sign a paper saying they understand the operation cannot be reversed.
	• If the wife dies or the couple divorce, then the man may marry another woman who wants children by him. He may be able to

have an operation to sew the vas together again. This is a more difficult operation and it can be expensive. Only half the men who have vasectomy reversed can have children after.

● Some men are frightened of operations. But a vasectomy is a very small operation.

● Some men think a vasectomy is the same as **castration**. They think they will lose their sexual power. If they talk to other men who have had a vasectomy they will discover it is not like this.

● The scrotum can swell up and become hot and painful. This is very rare but it needs medical treatment, so return to the hospital.

Female sterilization

What is female sterilization?

Female **sterilization** is a small operation to make a woman **sterile**, or unable to get pregnant. A woman can be sterilized if she has got all the children she wants, or there is a risk to her life if she becomes pregnant again.

How does sterilization work?

Each month an ovum is produced by an ovary inside the woman (see Chapter 2, page 21). This ovum travels along the fallopian tube. If the woman has sexual intercourse at this time, the ovum may be fertilized by a sperm.

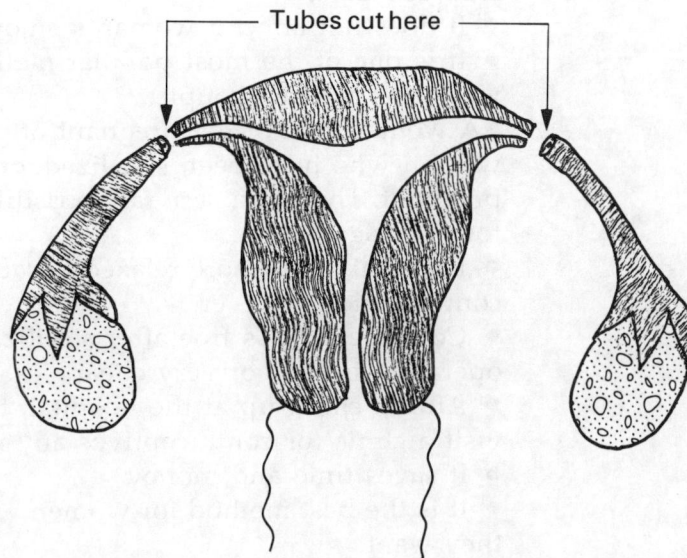

Female sterilization.

After discussing the operation with a doctor, the woman goes to a hospital or clinic. After a bath she is given an injection to make her fall asleep or she is given an injection in her back that stops her feeling any pain. The doctor cuts a small hole in her lower abdomen. He cuts the two fallopian tubes that carry the ovum to the uterus. Each tube end is tied to prevent them growing together again. Then he sews up the hole and the woman wakes up. The operation takes less than half an hour.

The woman has a sore abdomen for a few days while the cut heals. The stitches are removed after about five days. There will be a small scar on her abdomen. Some doctors cut the hole in the navel so that there is no scar.

The woman may go home after a few hours or she may be advised to stay in hospital for a few days for a good rest. She should not lift any heavy weights for at least a week. Aspirin or painkilling tablets will help to ease the sore abdomen.

The woman can have intercourse as soon as she feels ready, which may be in about two weeks. She should use a contraceptive until the first period after the operation. After that she never again need worry about pregnancy.

Advantages of sterilization

- There are no physical changes in a woman after sterilization. The woman has periods every month, but the ovum cannot reach the uterus.
- The ovaries continue to make female sex hormones, so she still feels **feminine**.
- It does not affect a woman's enjoyment or desire for sex.
- It is one of the most popular methods of contraception in the world for married couples.
- A woman cannot get pregnant after this operation. Out of 500 women who have been sterilized, only one woman will ever get pregnant. There is a *very* rare possibility that the tubes may grow together again.
- Lovemaking is more relaxed because a couple can forget about contraception for ever.
- Contraception is free after sterilization. In some countries the operation is free, or very cheap.
- After a check-up at the hospital, the woman does not have to visit a clinic for contraceptives any more.
- It saves time and money.
- It is the best method for women who have had all the children they want.
- It can be performed a few days after giving birth to a baby.
- Most women have the number of children they want by the time they are 30 years old, but they may be fertile for another 20 years.

- The operation is simple and can be performed in any hospital and many clinics.
- Apart from the doctor and husband, no-one knows that the woman has been sterilized, unless she tells them.

Disadvantages of sterilization

- It is not a method for unmarried women or young women.
- Sterilization is permanent. If the husband dies or the couple divorce, the woman may marry a man who wants more children. The woman may have an operation to sew the fallopian tubes together, but this is a longer and more difficult operation, and can only be done at special hospitals. Only half the women who have had their sterilizations reversed get pregnant later.
- The woman must rest for at least a week after the operation.
- There is a small chance of fever or infection. Any signs of fever, fainting, increasing pain or bleeding should be reported immediately to the hospital or clinic. Overweight or fat women are more at risk.
- Many women are frightened of this operation because they have heard untrue stories about it.
- Sterilization can only be performed by trained doctors or nurses in a hospital or clinic. A woman may have to travel some distance for the operation. But after that she is free from the worry of unwanted pregnancy.

> Sexual intercourse is like a juicy water melon, full of seeds. If the seeds are removed, the fruit is even nicer to eat. If the seeds of fertilization are removed as in male or female sterilization, then sexual intercourse is even better. The seeds or eggs do not get in the way of enjoyment.

New methods: Implants

What is an implant?

An **implant** is a tube of soft plastic 3 cm long and 2 mm thick. The implant is placed beneath the skin of a woman's upper arm. The implant contains contraceptive chemicals that are released into the bloodstream of the woman. The implant is left under the skin for up to five years and protects against pregnancy all that time.

How does the implant work?

The implant is inserted under the surface of the skin with a special **syringe** at a clinic. This is not painful. After 24 hours the woman is protected from pregnancy. After five years the implant is removed and a new one inserted.

The chemicals are released from the implant at the same rate as taking one contraceptive pill a day. The implant works like the Mini-Pill. Ovulation stops and the cervical mucus becomes extra thick which prevents sperm travelling into the uterus.

Advantages of implants

- They are a safe and reliable contraceptive for most women of all ages.
- Out of 100 women using implants for ten years, only one will get pregnant.
- Women can forget about contraception for five years.
- No-one knows if a woman is using the implant.
- If the woman wants to have a baby, the implant can be easily removed at a clinic. The effect wears off after 24 hours.
- A woman's fertility is not affected when she stops using the implant.

Disadvantages of implants

- The implant must be fitted by trained health workers.
- Some women have irregular periods with the implant.
- Some women have no periods for a few months, so they may worry that they are pregnant.
- Implants are a new contraceptive so they are not yet available everywhere.

New methods: The sponge

What is the sponge?

The sponge is a circle of soft plastic foam containing spermicide that is inserted into the vagina. The sponge is shaped to fit over the cervix and has a ribbon to pull it out of the vagina after use.

How does the sponge work?

The spermicide in the sponge destroys sperm after intercourse and the sponge prevents sperm from entering the uterus.

How is the sponge used?

The sponge is wetted with clean water and then inserted to the top of the vagina with the finger. The woman cannot feel the sponge inside her and it cannot get lost. It can be inserted 24 hours before or a few minutes before intercourse. The sponge is left inside for at least six hours, or up to 24 hours after lovemaking.

Advantages of the sponge

- It can be bought in pharmacies without visiting a clinic.
- It does not affect a woman's menstrual cycle or her health.
- The couple can have intercourse several times in 24 hours without changing the sponge.

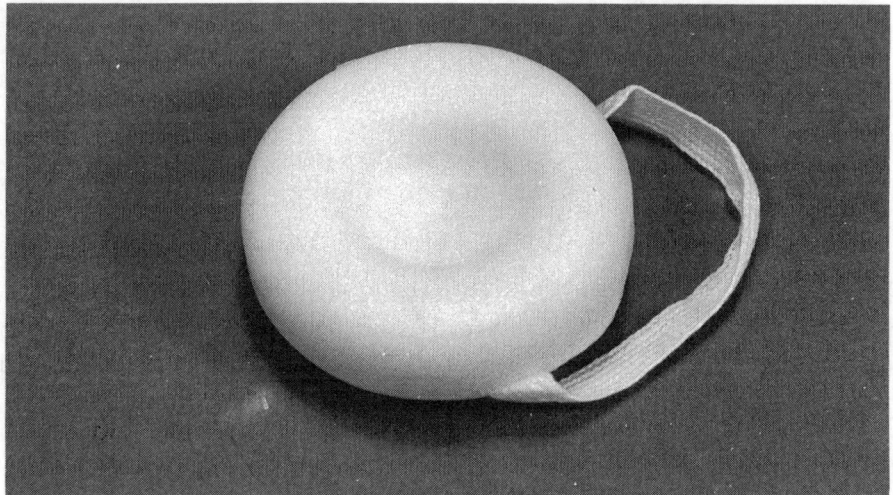

The sponge.

Disadvantages of the sponge

- It is not a reliable method of contraception. It is safer than using nothing, but other methods such as the condom or cap are better. The sponge is only suitable for women who do not mind if they get pregnant.
- Out of 100 women using the sponge for a year, 15 to 25 may become pregnant.
- It can be pushed out of place by the penis, which would allow sperm into the uterus.
- The spermicide may irritate the delicate skin of the vagina.
- If it is left inside for longer than 24 hours, infection can occur.
- Each sponge can only be used once.
- It is more expensive than other contraceptives.

Emergency sponge

If you are a long way from a clinic or pharmacy this method is better than nothing in preventing pregnancy.

You need either a round sea sponge or a plastic foam sponge about 5 cm by 5 cm. If you have no sponge, then use cotton, kapok or soft cloth.

1 Mix 2 large spoons of vinegar in 1 cup of clean water

OR

1 small spoon of lemon juice in 1 cup of clean water

OR

1 spoon of salt in 4 spoons of clean water

2 Wet the sponge with one of these mixtures.

3 Push the wet sponge to the top of the vagina before having intercourse. You can put it in up to an hour before.

4 After intercourse leave the sponge in for at least 6 hours,

111

but not more than 12 hours. Take it out. Wash the sponge and dry it in the sun. Throw away the cotton or kapok.

This method should only be used in an emergency when nothing else is available.

If 100 couples used this method for a year about 30 women could get pregnant.

Post-coital (after-sex) contraception

This is contraception that is used after sex when no contraceptives were used, but the woman does not want to be pregnant. After-sex contraception prevents conception, even if it does not prevent fertilization. Conception occurs when the fertilized ovum starts to grow in the uterus, some days after fertilization between the sperm and ovum.

There are two after-sex methods:

1 Intra-Uterine Device method

A copper-covered IUD is inserted into the uterus. This can be done up to nine days before the expected day of the woman's next period. This prevents pregnancy even if there have been several acts of sex without contraception.

2 Combined Pill method

Two tablets of a high dose contraceptive Pill are taken *not more than 72 hours* after sex without contraception. This is followed by a further two tablets exactly 12 hours later. Not any contraceptive Pill will work — the correct type must be used. The woman must take the tablets *exactly* as instructed. This method will not prevent pregnancy if the woman has further sex without contraception. She must use another method, such as a condom, or start taking the contraceptive Pill regularly.

How does it work?

Both methods prevent a fertilized ovum from growing in the uterus, so that it comes away with the next period. This is not abortion, so is therefore legal. The Combined Pill method may prevent ovulation, so that fertilization would not occur. These methods have to be used as soon as possible after sex without contraception. The woman must be sure she is not already pregnant.

The woman must be completely honest with the clinic about the dates of her last period, and the dates and number of times she has had sex without contraception. The nurse or doctor will need to examine her to ensure she is not already some weeks pregnant. If there is any pain in the abdomen, or unusual bleeding after treatment the woman must return to the clinic immediately. Further sex without contraception must be avoided.

After-sex contraception may be needed when:
• Intercourse was not expected, so the couple had no contraceptives.

- The couple were under the influence of alcohol or drugs.
- The couple did not understand how to use the Natural Method and had intercourse during the fertile days.
- The woman was raped.
- The woman had taken medicines or had a disease, such as rubella, that could harm a foetus.
- A condom split or slipped off during intercourse.
- The woman forgot to take her contraceptive pills for a whole week and did not use a condom instead.
- The diaphragm was inserted incorrectly, or moved.

Advantages of after-sex contraception

- After-sex contraception can prevent an unwanted pregnancy in an emergency.
- If the IUD method is used, then the IUD can remain inside the woman's uterus. If she wishes to use another method of contraception, then she can have the IUD removed after her next period.
- Both methods are very reliable. For every 100 women who use them, only two will get pregnant.

Disadvantages of after-sex contraception

- After-sex contraception must always be given by a clinic.
- There is an important time limit. The IUD method must be used nine days before the next expected period, or up to five days after ovulation. The Combined Pill method must be used within three days of unprotected sex.
- There is a very small risk that if pregnancy still occurs after using after-sex contraception, there could be problems. With the IUD the pregnancy could be **ectopic**. Not enough research has been done to know if a baby could be harmed by the Combined Pill method.
- After-sex contraception is for emergencies only: it should not be used regularly. The large hormonal dose is more than a woman would take in a month if she took the Pill every day.
- The clinic must be sure that the woman is not already pregnant from previous sex without contraception.
- After-sex contraception is not yet understood by all child spacing clinics.
- The Combined Pill method is less effective if there have been several acts of sex without contraception.
- With the Combined Pill method most women feel nauseous for 12 to 36 hours. Some women vomit, feel dizzy or have headaches.
- Some women should not use the Combined Pill method. This does not apply to older women, or women with high blood pressure, for whom pregnancy would be even more dangerous.
- Pain may be felt at insertion of the IUD, or afterwards.
- If there is existing pelvic infection, the insertion of an IUD could increase it.

Breastfeeding

Breastfeeding is good for babies. It is also used by many mothers to space their children. This can be effective for some women, but not for all.

How does breastfeeding work?

Many women have no periods while they are breastfeeding. When the baby sucks on the nipple, hormones are sent to the ovaries to stop ovulation (see Chapter 2, page 21). If the baby is not breastfed for some hours, ovulation may occur and a period will appear 14 days later. If the mother breastfeeds at least every two hours in the day and every four hours at night, and the baby receives only breast milk, then she may not have periods. When the baby breastfeeds less often and eats other foods, ovulation and periods begin. Even if only a few breastfeeds are missed, a woman can get pregnant. But a woman cannot know when her periods are going to start, so she may get pregnant before her first period. If the baby is bottle fed, or only breastfed during the day, the mother's periods will start sooner. Some women begin periods four weeks after birth.

Once a woman has had one period after the birth, she may get pregnant as easily as she did before. A woman should not stop breastfeeding when her periods begin, but she must use a contraceptive to space her children.

All women should use contraceptives within three months of giving birth, and within one month of birth if not breastfeeding.

If the mother wants another child she should try to wait for three years so the first baby has time to get strong (see page 75).

What contraceptive is most suitable while breastfeeding?

● Condoms, caps and spermicides are safe during breastfeeding. They cannot affect the milk. The cap should be checked after childbirth as the vagina may change shape after a birth (see page 91).

● IUDs can be used, but they may fall out if inserted too soon after a birth. The mother may feel some discomfort while breastfeeding as the uterus contracts around the IUD (see page 88).

● Sterilization can be performed immediately after birth on mothers who are sure they have completed their families. The baby can continue to breastfeed in hospital with the mother (see page 107).

● The Pill is often given to breastfeeding mothers. The high dose Combined Pill may reduce the amount of milk produced. Little is known about the possible effects on the baby if some of the contraceptive passes into the milk. The low dose Mini-Pill does not affect the milk supply and is safer for the baby. Remember the Mini-Pill must be taken at the same time each day (see page 81). Start the Pill four weeks after birth.

● Dep-Provera injectables do not affect the milk supply and

sometimes increase it. The first injection should be given four weeks after birth.

> Breastfeeding is best for babies for at least two years
> but
> it is not a completely reliable contraceptive method.

Abortion

Abortion is not a contraceptive method. Abortion is an operation to end an unwanted pregnancy before a baby is ready to be born. Abortion is a dangerous operation unless it is performed by doctors in a hospital. Illegal or **backstreet abortions** are a major cause of death among women in some countries. Nobody should ever have an abortion performed by an untrained person. In most countries, abortion is against the law. Any person who helps a woman to abort may be imprisoned. The woman too may face punishment.

Backstreet abortions are always dangerous, painful and expensive. They are done in unclean places using dirty instruments. The abortionist may pour acids or poisons or push sharp sticks or objects into the uterus. The woman may drink poisonous herbs or drugs.

These methods may end the pregnancy, but more often they also cause heavy bleeding, infection and damage to the uterus. The woman may still be pregnant, but the growing foetus may be damaged or deformed. Parts of the dead foetus may be left inside and start to go rotten. This causes heavy bleeding, blood poisoning and death. Even if the infection is cured the woman may be sterile and unable to have children later when she wants them.

> Backstreet abortions are always dangerous.
> The only safe abortion is in hospital, early in pregnancy.

The complications of illegal abortions include:
- Heavy bleeding.
- Blood poisoning.
- Tetanus.   } can cause the death of the
- Fever.   woman
- Damage to the intestines.
- Damage to the uterus.   } can cause infertility
- Infection.
- Damage to the foetus.

The arguments for and against legal abortion are mostly about

115

when the life of a person begins. Is it at conception, during pregnancy, or at birth? Is a small foetus already a human? Is the abortion of a foetus the same as the murder of a child? These are difficult questions that scientists and religious leaders are still discussing.

Many people believe that all abortion is murder. Others believe that the mother's life is more important and that she should have control over her own body. Abortion is a sad solution to a difficult problem. But safe, legal abortions are better then dangerous, backstreet abortions.

Different religions have different beliefs. Catholic Christians are against all abortions and most methods of contraception. Some Protestant Christians accept abortion at an early stage if the mother's mental or physical health is at risk. The Jewish faith allows abortion as they believe that the foetus is part of the mother and not a separate person. The Islamic faith allows abortion up to 17 weeks. Hindus allow abortion only when the mother's life is in danger.

Whatever the laws or beliefs of a country, many thousands of women with unwanted pregnancies still choose an abortion. They may try to abort themselves, or they may go to an abortionist. Rich women may seek an abortion in another country. Poor women have dangerous backstreet abortions and often die. If couples use contraceptives they can prevent unwanted pregnancies and avoid the need for abortions.

Legal abortions

In some countries abortion is legal. Women cannot demand abortions, but doctors are permitted to perform them.

An abortion may be given if:
- A woman is sick and being pregnant could put her life in danger.
- The pregnancy is in the fallopian tube and not in the uterus. This would kill the woman.
- The foetus is known to be deformed.
- The woman has been raped.
- The couple have been using contraception but the method failed. No contraception is 100% reliable, except for sterilization.
- A girl is still at school or college and the father will not support her and the baby.
- The woman has several other children who would suffer from having an extra child to feed in the family.

In these cases, a doctor may give a woman an abortion if the woman herself feels it is right. Young girls will usually need their parent's agreement.

A woman who needs an abortion must talk to her doctor as soon as she misses one period. Pregnancy will not go away by itself. An abortion is safest if it is performed in hospital before 12 weeks of pregnancy, but it may be expensive. There may be a long waiting list. The hospital will be busy with other operations and there may not be enough doctors to perform the abortion.

Abortion is a difficult decision. Nobody should be forced to have an abortion. But if a woman chooses to have one, she needs support. Abortion is usually an unnecessary operation. Most abortions can be prevented if the couple uses contraceptives.

> Prevent abortions — use contraceptives.

Methods of abortion in hospital

Legal abortions are performed in germ-free hospitals or clinics by trained nurses and doctors.

- Up to 12 weeks of a pregnancy

A narrow plastic tube is inserted up the vagina and into the uterus. The other end of the tube is attached to a machine which sucks out the embryo and placenta. The woman may be asleep or awake. She can go home after a few hours. This is called **suction evacuation**.

- Up to 16 weeks of pregnancy

The woman is put to sleep and the cervix is stretched open. The foetus and the placenta are scraped out through the vagina, with a special instrument. The woman stays in hospital for a night. This is called dilatation and extraction.

- After 16 weeks of pregnancy

The foetus and placenta are too large to scrape out. The woman is given an injection often into the womb, or a pessary in the vagina. This makes the uterus contract, as in birth. The woman is awake and given painkillers. After a few hours the foetus and placenta come out of the vagina. An abortion at 20 weeks is like a birth — the foetus looks like a small baby, but cannot live. Late abortions are less safe for the woman. Abortion may be legal up to about 24 weeks, depending on the country.

After an abortion most women bleed as if they were having a light period, for up to two weeks. Some women feel relieved after an abortion. Other women feel sad, depressed, angry or guilty, even though they chose an abortion. After an abortion, a woman needs support from her health workers, friends or family.

Even after abortions in hospital, some women may have problems. If any of these danger signs occur after an abortion, go straight to a clinic.

- Fever.
- Heavy bleeding.
- Passing piece of meat-like material from the vagina.

117

- Light bleeding for more than three weeks.
- Severe pain in the abdomen.
- Smelly discharge from the vagina.
- Weakness or muscle aches.
- Cramps or backache.
- No periods six weeks after the abortion.

Non – methods of contraception

Many people believe the following prevent pregnancy. They do not.

Myth: Making love standing up or with the woman on top.
Truth: Sperm can easily swim upwards.

Myth: Making love in the sea, a bath, a river or a shower.
Truth: The vagina fits tightly around the penis during intercourse so that water will not wash away the sperm.

Myth: Making love during a menstrual period.
Truth: Sperm can swim through menstrual flow. There may be an early ovum in the fallopian tube, waiting to be fertilized.

Myth: The woman urinates immediately after intercourse.
Truth: The vagina and the urethra are not connected. Urine comes out through the urethra, so it will not wash away the sperm in the vagina.

Myth: The woman is a virgin.
Truth: If the man ejaculates in or near the vagina, a pregnancy can occur. Even if a woman is a virgin, there is still a small hole for the sperm to swim up into the vagina.

Myth: The woman has only just started having periods.
Truth: Any woman who has periods, or is about to start having periods can get pregnant.

Myth: The woman does not have an orgasm.
Truth: The orgasm of a woman has little effect on conception. If the ovum is ready, and the sperm are there, then she will get pregnant.

Myth: The woman jumps up and down, coughs or sneezes after intercourse.
Truth: The uterus can hold the sperm inside the woman for several days, whatever the woman does.

Myth:	The woman has a hot bath.
Truth:	The hole through the cervix is too small for water to pass through, but big enough for sperm. A hot bath will not wash out the sperm.

Myth:	The man squeezes his testicles during or before ejaculating.
Truth:	The sperm will still come out with the semen. The sperm ducts are very narrow and cannot be squeezed shut. The sperm start to travel towards the penis before ejaculation.

> None of these methods work.
> Use contraceptives to prevent pregnancy.

Dear Auntie,

My sister told me that if I got pregnant by mistake I could cause an abortion by eating a box of washing powder. Does this work?

Hannah

Dear Hannah,

No, it certainly does not work! Eating a box of washing powder would make you very sick. Even if you did manage to eat the washing powder, which would be very difficult, it would not cause you to abort the pregnancy. The mouth and the uterus are not connected, so the washing powder could not wash out the uterus in the same way that it washes your clothes.

Putting washing powder into the vagina or uterus is also very dangerous. The chemicals in the powder could cause poisoning, infection, infertility or death.

Never try to stop an unwanted pregnancy by drinking poisons or sticking things up the vagina. In many countries this is illegal, and you may die. If you live in a country where abortion is allowed, go and visit a doctor as soon as you think you may be pregnant. If the doctor agrees you need an abortion, he can arrange for a safe operation in a hospital.

Dear Auntie,

Last year I slept with a girl who is now pregnant. She says I am the father, but I know that she also slept with other men. Is there any way I can prove that I am not the father?

Michael

Dear Michael,

Yes, it is possible. Tests can compare your blood group with the baby's and the mother's blood group. If your blood is a different group from the baby's and the mother's, then you cannot be the father. But if the baby's blood group is the same as yours, then you *may* be the father. If all the men involved had the same blood group as each other, and the baby, then the father could be any one of you!

In future, don't have sex with anyone unless you use a contraceptive, and you are willing to accept the responsibility of a pregnancy. Pregnancy is as much the responsibility of the man as the woman. Sex always carries a risk unless you are married.

Activities

1 What is the purpose of child spacing? Find out how many children there are in each family in your community. How many years are there between each child?

2 Plant some radish or cabbage seeds very close to each other in the soil. Plant some more further apart. Water them every day. Which plants grow best?

3 Make up a role-play about a family with lots of children and another family with well spaced children.

4 Discuss contraception and young people. Do you think contraceptives should be available to unmarried people? What are the advantages and disadvantages?

5 Most societies have traditional methods of birth control. What methods are used in your society? Do they work?

6 Ask a local health worker to demonstrate methods of contraception to the group. Discuss each method's advantages and disadvantages.

7 Draw a poster about child spacing and its benefits. Find out the times that your local child spacing clinic is open and include this on the poster.

Quiz

1 Put the following contraceptive methods in order of effectiveness:

a) The Pill; b) Natural methods; c) IUD; d) Condom; e) Cap;
f) Withdrawal.

2 Match the following contraceptives with their advantages:
a) The Pill; b) IUD; c) Condom; d) Natural methods.

1) Easily available from shops; 2) Effective prevention of pregnancy; 3) Approved by the Catholic Church; 4) Requires few visits to clinic.

3 Match the following contraceptives with their disadvantages:
a) The Pill; b) IUD; c) Condom; d) Natural methods.

1) Can cause heavy periods; 2) Good understanding of menstrual cycle needed; 3) Can interrupt lovemaking; 4) Unsuitable for older women.

4 When a man has a vasectomy he: a) has a normal erection;
b) can have a good sex life; c) has no sperm in his semen; d) can never make a woman pregnant.

1) a, d, e, c, b, f.
2) a-2; b-4; c-1; d-3.
3) a-4; b-1; c-3; d-2.
4) All are true.

CHAPTER 6
Sexually transmitted diseases

A sexually transmitted disease, or STD is the same as a venereal disease, or VD. The term 'sexually transmitted disease' covers several diseases, which can be caught by close physical contact with an infected person. Sexual intercourse is the usual way of spreading any STD.

Everyone catches infections of some kind during their lives. Sexual infections are not always worse than many kinds of diseases, such as measles or tetanus. But some of them can seriously damage the body if not treated. And they can be passed on to other people without their knowing about it.

Anyone can catch an STD by having sex with just one person who is infected. An STD can be caught by someone who has only slept with one partner in their life, if that partner has slept with another infected person. But the more partners a person has, the

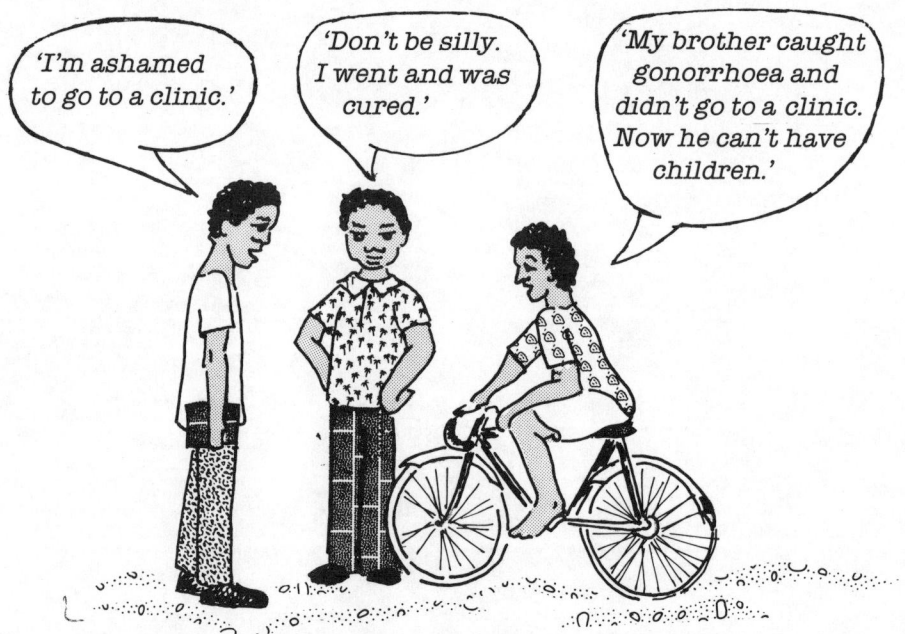

'I'm ashamed to go to a clinic.'

'Don't be silly. I went and was cured.'

'My brother caught gonorrhoea and didn't go to a clinic. Now he can't have children.'

Do not be ashamed to go to a clinic.

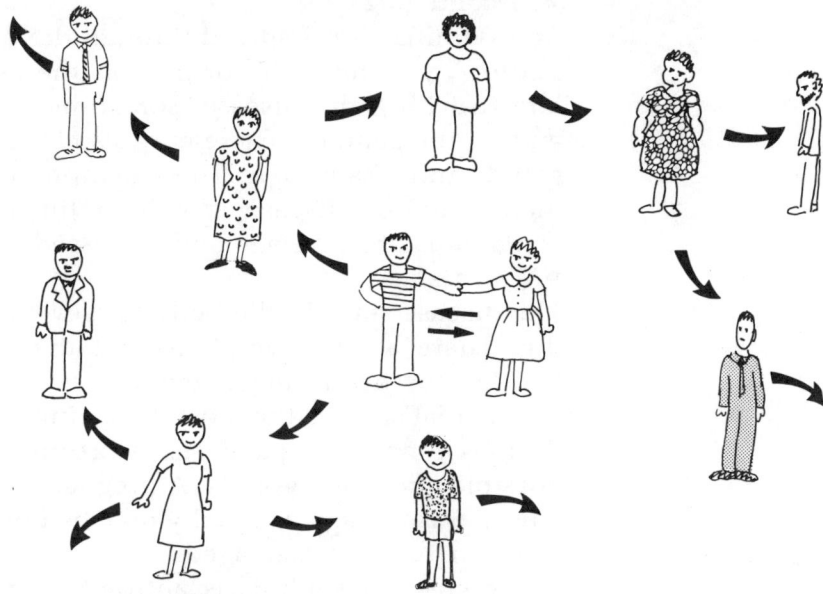

The spread of STDs.

greater the risk of catching an STD. Some of these diseases can sleep in the body for several months before any symptoms appear. So even if a couple have been faithful to each other for a long time, one of them could start getting symptoms.

STDs are connected with guilt, fear, shame, silence and ignorance — which helps them to spread further. If more people knew about the symptoms and would admit to having an STD, then the diseases would not spread so fast. But many people feel guilty about having an STD and do not tell their partners. The partner may then pass the disease to someone else, or back to their treated partner. The only way to be safe from catching an STD is to have sex with one partner, who also only has sex with you.

Syphilis, also called the pox, or bad blood

Syphilis takes many years to damage the body. The disease usually has three stages.
● First stage
A hard painless sore appears on the genitals about three to six weeks after contact with an infected partner. If the sore is inside the anus or vagina it may not be noticed, so a woman may not realise she has syphilis. After a few weeks the sores go away without treatment. But the disease stays in the body. Syphilis can be detected by looking at the pus from the sore under a microscope. When there are no sores a blood test will reveal the disease.

• Second stage

The syphilis germs spread through the blood to every part of the body. A general rash appears on the skin, seven to ten weeks after catching the disease, sometimes with sores in the mouth and on the genitals. There may also be fever, sore throat, swollen glands and loss of hair. These symptoms go away without treatment, but the disease is still in the body. Syphilis is highly **contagious** at this stage and is passed on to all partners.

• Third stage

The disease stays in the body for several years before re-appearing. There are no symptoms but the disease is damaging the body — the heart, lungs, genitals, eyes, nervous system, brain.

The final stage is the most damaging. Brain damage, blindness, deafness, madness, paralysis, heart disease and infertility are all possible effects of syphilis. A pregnant woman with syphilis may have a miscarriage. Her baby may be born dead, or die soon after birth, or be brain damaged.

The cure for syphilis is antibiotic injections. Syphilis can be cured at any stage, but damaged parts of the body cannot be repaired. Early treatment is needed to prevent permanent damage to the body.

Gonorrhoea, also called the clap or dose

Gonorrhoea is the most common STD known, and very infectious. The gonorrhoea germ can only live inside the body and dies after a few seconds in the air. The gonorrhoea germ enters the body through the wet parts — vulva, glans, urethra, mouth, eyes.

The symptoms of gonorrhoea may appear from two to ten days after having sex with an infected partner.

• In a man:
— Yellow or white pus leaking from the penis.
— Burning feeling with urinating.
— Itching or pain in penis.

• In a woman:
— Yellow or white discharge from vagina.
— Burning feeling when urinating.
— Sometimes a fever, or pains in stomach and joints of bones.

Most women have no symptoms. Even if there are no symptoms the woman must be treated if her partner is infected. If gonorrhoea is not treated then the germs can spread to the reproductive parts. The tubes become blocked with inflammation and scars. This causes infertility in a woman or man, and blockage of the man's urethra so he cannot urinate. A baby can be blinded if born to a woman with gonorrhoea — the gonorrhoea gets into the baby's eyes as it is born.

Gonorrhoea is treated with antibiotics, by injection or tablets.

There are other minor complaints that are not strictly STDs, but can be caught from close physical or sexual contact. They are dealt with below.

Genital herpes

There are many different types of **herpes.** The most common type of herpes is the cold sore that appears on the lips. Genital herpes is similar, but appears on the genitals. About two to 14 days after contact with the herpes, small blisters appear. They are painful or itchy. They fill with clear or yellow liquid. The blister breaks and leaves a raw sore which takes two to three weeks to heal. Herpes sores may cause discomfort when urinating. Bathe the sores in one litre of warm water and two teaspoons of salt, four times a day. Keep the sores dry and do not let your clothes rub against them. Wear loose cotton pants. Always wash the hands with soap and water after touching the sores. Do not share towels or washing cloths. The sores usually heal in one or two weeks. Sometimes there are painful lumps at the top of the leg. Symptoms such as headache, backache, or a fever may sometimes come with the sores.

Herpes is very infectious when the sores are visible. Once the disease starts the sores may re-appear for no reason. Some people never get another attack after the first one. There is no treatment and anyone with herpes should not have sexual contact while they have sores. Herpes can affect babies as they are being born.

Genital warts

These look like ordinary **warts**, but appear on the genitals anything from one to nine months after infection. They should be treated as soon as possible or they will grow larger and spread to other people.

Chancroid

Chancroid appears as a painful sore on the penis or vulva (unlike syphilis, which are painless). At the same time or before the sores appear, the glands at the top of the leg become swollen. Chancroid is more common in men but more serious for women. Chancroid is sometimes confused with syphilis and genital herpes. It can be cured with antibiotics. If not treated the sores spread and swell seriously in the genitals.

Cystitis or honeymoon bladder

Cystitis is very common in women but it is not usually due to infection from the partner. Cystitis is not usually a dangerous disease, but it can be very unpleasant. The woman's urethra is very short so germs can easily get from the urethra and into the

125

bladder. Women sometimes develop inflammation of the bladder after having sex for the first time, or after energetic lovemaking. Cystitis can be caused by bruising of the bladder by the penis through the walls of the vagina.

The main symptom of cystitis is the need to urinate often, with a burning pain and very little urine. Other possible symptoms are fever, an ache in the lower abdomen or back, and cloudy urine. If there is any pain or bleeding, then visit a clinic. In a bad case of cystitis, the inflammation can spread to the kidneys and damage them. The treatment is antibiotic tablets.

The following will help if cystitis starts:
- Drink a large glass of water every 20 minutes. Add one tea-spoon of bicarbonate of soda (baking powder) once an hour. This tastes horrible, but will help reduce the burning and pain.
- Drink at least 3 litres of water, milk, weak tea or weak orange squash every day. The bladder needs lots of liquids to wash out the germs.
- Go to the toilet at least six times a day (you may want to anyway!)
- Wash the vulva with warm water after each visit to the toilet. Do not use strong soap, antiseptic or cream. Use a clean cloth and do not share it with anyone else.
- Rubber bottles filled with hot water will ease the pain. Hold them on the lower back or between the legs.
- Rest as much as possible.
- Do not drink any alcohol until the cystitis clears up.

After three hours of this routine the cystitis may have eased.
- Go to the clinic if
— The cystitis lasts more than two days.
— You are pregnant.
— There is blood in the urine.
— Cystitis occurs in men or children.

Some women have sensitive bladders and suffer from repeated attacks of cystitis. You can help to prevent further attacks by drinking at least two litres of water every day. Go to the toilet whenever you feel the need: do not wait. Make sure that the bladder is properly emptied.

Avoid drinking tea, coffee or alcohol, or make them weaker. Follow the instructions for avoiding vaginal infections on the facing page.

If cystitis often occurs after sexual intercourse then tell your partner. Both partners should wash their genitals before inter-course and dry them gently. Use a lubricant during intercourse to prevent soreness and bruising. The woman should go to the toilet 15 minutes before intercourse and within 15 minutes after intercourse. Make love gently.

126

Vaginal infections

The vagina produces discharge to keep it moist and healthy. With a vaginal infection the discharge may smell unpleasant and be thick and dark yellow, white, grey or pale green. The vagina becomes very itchy. A vaginal infection is not always a sexually transmitted disease. Vaginal infections are more common when women are over tired, anaemic, upset or taking the Pill.

If a woman thinks she may have a vaginal infection such as thrush, vaginitis or urethritis she should visit the clinic. Meanwhile she can help herself with the following:
- Keep the vagina as dry as possible.
- Stop using soap on the vulva. Wash with water only.
- Do not scratch — this only makes it worse.
- Check that there is no tampon left inside the vagina.
- Do not have sex, unless a condom is used.
- Finish the treatment. Do not stop when the symptoms go.
- Tell all your partners. They may need treatment too. Vaginal infections can be carried by men without any symptoms. They occasionally cause inflammation of the penis.

Preventing vaginal infections

- Wear cotton pants or no pants. Do not wear nylon pants, tights or tight trousers.
- Wear clean pants every day.
- Do not use deodorants, disinfectants or perfumed soap on the vulva. These all irritate the sensitive skin.
- Always wash and wipe the vulva from front to back. This prevents any germs from the faeces entering the vagina.
- Avoid antibiotics unless really necessary. Antibiotics can encourage vaginal infections by destroying 'good' germs.

Non-specific vaginitis or NSV

Any infection which has symptoms, but tests cannot show exactly which germs are involved, is called 'non-specific.' '-itis' means an infection in that part of the body. Any unusual discharge from the vagina which may be white, yellow, green, grey or blood streaked should be reported to a clinic. The first sign of an infection may be pain or burning when urinating. Vaginitis can be caught from an infected partner, but not always. Treatment is with pessary tablets inserted in the vagina and cream.

Non-specific urethritis or NSU

Any infection of the genitals or urinary system that cannot be identified by tests is called 'non-specific'. **Urethritis** is even more common than gonorrhoea. It is usually spread by sexual contact, but not always.

The symptoms are discharge from the penis and pain or burning when urinating. Men often catch urethritis at the same time

127

as catching gonorrhoea. Different medicines are needed to treat each disease. Treatment for urethritis is with antibiotic tablets.

Thrush, or yeast infection

Thrush usually occurs only in women. It is caused by yeast germs which live normally on the skin. The vagina becomes very itchy and there is a thick white discharge that smells like baking bread. The vulva may swell and be sore. Urinating may be painful. Mothers with thrush must wash their hands after going to the toilet as thrush can infect a baby's eyes. Treatment is with cream and pessary tablets that are inserted into the vagina. Antibiotics can make thrush worse. Thrush is more common in pregnant women.

Treatment of STDs

If you have any symptoms that *may* be an STD, then visit a clinic *today* not tomorrow.

> The sooner an STD is treated, the quicker it will be cured.

Main symptoms of STDs:
- Any spots or sores, lumps or swellings, rash or itching on or near the genitals.
- Any discharge from the penis.
- Unusual discharge from the vagina.
- Pain or burning when urinating.

Never try to forget about a discharge or sores. STDs never go away without treatment. The symptoms may go away for a while, but the disease stays in the body. The symptoms of STDs may be similar to other diseases. The disease will be damaging the body even though there is no pain. Pretending not to have the disease means that the patients, their partners and their children will suffer. Or they may never be able to have children.

Go to a clinic for treatment, if possible with your partner. Some places have Special STD Clinics, other places treat all diseases at the same clinic. The health workers at Special Clinics are trained to treat STDs. They are helpful and understanding towards all patients attending a Special Clinic. To find a clinic, look at posters in toilets or beer halls or health centres or post offices. Ask at the local health centre or telephone a doctor. You do not need an appointment, or a letter from your doctor.

In some countries treatment for STDs is free from government clinics and hospitals. The cost of treatment is always less than the cost of damaging the body, or someone else's body.

Never try and treat an STD yourself. Always go to a clinic. If you are embarrassed about visiting the local clinic, then go to one further away from home. No-one in the clinic will tell anyone else.

The clinic will ask for your name and address. This will not be passed on to anyone else. The clinic may give you a number so that your name is kept secret. The clinic knows that if they do not treat their patients kindly, they will not return for all the treatment.

The clinic will ask several questions about your life. Telling the truth is important. The health worker needs to know about:
- Your symptoms, for example sores or burning urine.
- How long the symptoms have lasted.
- The type of sex the patient has had, for example oral or anal sex.
- Allergy to any drugs or medicines.
- If a woman patient is, or may be pregnant. This is because some medicines may affect an unborn baby.

The health worker will examine the genitals. A sample of the discharge is taken from the penis or vagina and examined under a microscope. A urine sample and a small blood sample is examined under a microscope. This does not hurt. You will be asked how many sex partners you have had in the past three months (or longer if the symptoms have lasted for longer). Honesty is important so that all the partners can be contacted and treated too. The clinic will not tell the partners who told them. They may have printed cards to give or send to partners. The card tells them they must visit a clinic as soon as possible for treatment. If you do not want to tell the clinic who your partners have been, then you must tell them yourself. If you do not they may pass the disease back to you, or to someone else. They could become seriously ill or become infertile, or die.

If the patient has an STD then the clinic will prescribe the correct medicine needed to treat that disease. There are many types of medicines and different antibiotics. Each disease needs a different dose and type of medicine. Because of misuse, some diseases cannot be cured by certain medicines. New medicines are invented to overcome this resistance. If you have a **resistant** form of the disease, the clinic may ask you to return for more treatment. Do not refuse. Every time someone is not treated properly, it makes the disease stronger and more difficult to treat next time.

During treatment for STDs remember:
- Never have sex with anyone while the disease is being treated, even if the partner is also being treated. Wait until the clinic says the disease is completely cured.
- Both partners must finish the treatment. For gonorrhoea this

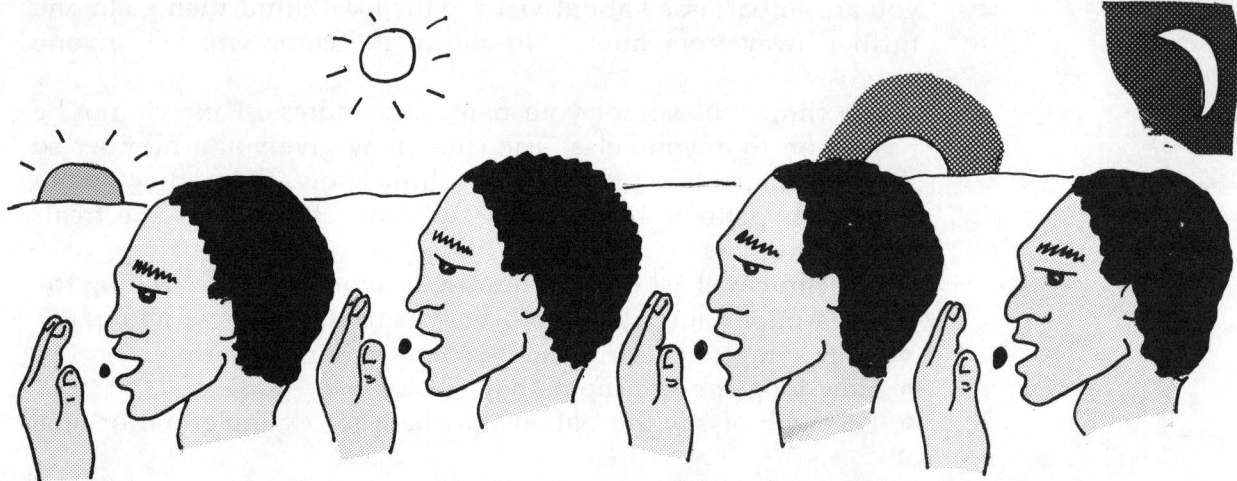

Take tablets throughout the day.

may be daily injections of antibiotics for five days. For syphilis the treatment may be longer. Although antibiotic tablets work just as well, some clinics prefer to give injections. They fear that some patients may forget to take all the tablets, or give them away.

- If not enough tablets are taken then the sores or discharge may go away, but the disease will stay in the body. A small dose is like cutting off the top of a weed above the ground. The roots are still there and will grow again, possibly even stronger. Diseases such as gonorrhoea, have grown stronger and resistant over the years because the disease was only half treated.
- Take the medicines exactly as the clinic describes. 'One tablet every 8 hours' does *not* mean 3 tablets once a day.
- Never take more of the medicine than the clinic prescribes. A cure is not quicker by taking all the medicine at once, or in a shorter time. Medicine needs time to work.
- Never take someone else's treatment. Each person needs a different dose.
- Never buy treatment from a market, street seller, or friends. They do not know the correct dose and the medicine may be out of date. Out of date antibiotics are dangerous — they can make a disease worse.
- Never drink alcohol or take drugs while being treated for STDs. Mixing alcohol or drugs with antibiotics can make a person very ill, or stop the medicine from treating the disease.

Always finish a course of treatment.

130

Once an STD is cured, anyone can catch an STD again if they have sex with someone who is infected.

There is no immunity to STDs.

STDs are only dangerous when they remain untreated secrets. If everyone who ever caught an STD was treated quickly before they passed it to someone else, then the diseases would disappear. People should not feel guilty about catching an STD. But they should feel guilty if they pass the disease to someone else because they did not get treated.

Anyone who thinks they may have an STD should do the following:

- Stop having sex with anyone, even their husband or wife.
- Go to a clinic or doctor immediately for treatment.
- Tell all their sexual partners − either by word or by letter.
- Try not to catch or spread an STD again.

Preventing STDs   Know your partner well enough to be able to trust him or her. Many STDs are caught from 'friends' who are not honest enough to admit that they may have a disease.

Do not have sex with anyone who has any inflammation, sore

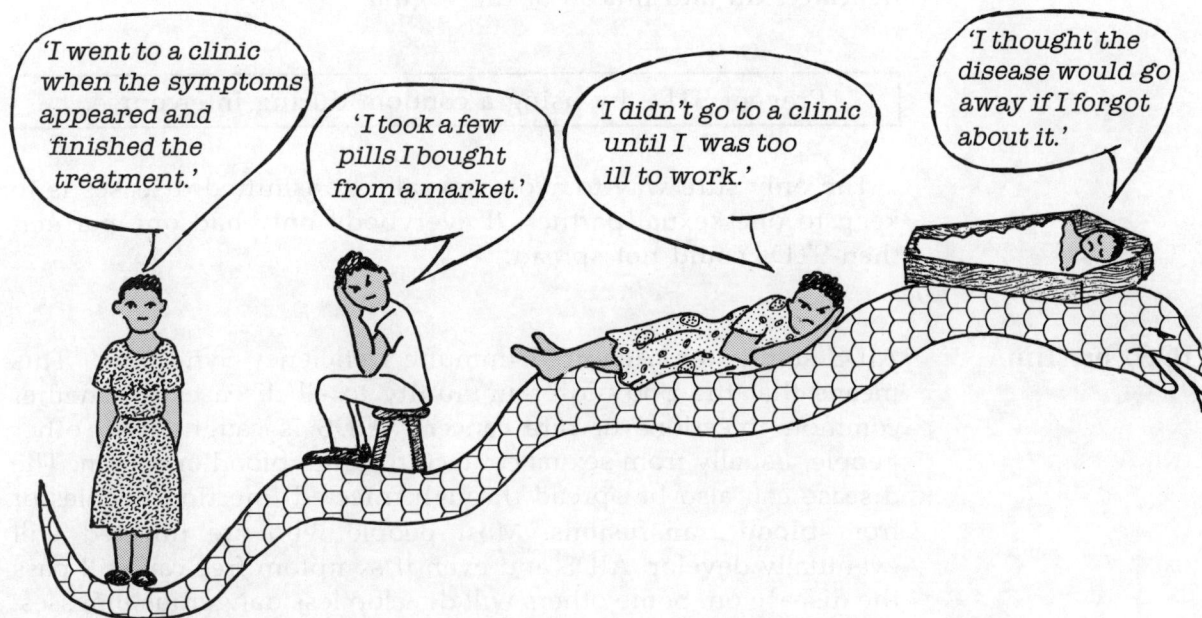

'I went to a clinic when the symptoms appeared and finished the treatment.'

'I took a few pills I bought from a market.'

'I didn't go to a clinic until I was too ill to work.'

'I thought the disease would go away if I forgot about it.'

Do not give STDs the chance to become strong.

or unusual discharge around the genital area. Suggest that they visit a clinic.

Keep to one partner whom you know. Changing partners or having several at once is an easy way of catching an STD. The best prevention is to wait until marriage, and then remain faithful to each other.

Think before having sex.

Condoms help to prevent the spread of gonorrhoea and AIDS. This is not a guaranteed prevention. If you know your partner has a disease, then do not sleep together.

Both men and women should:
- Wash all around genitals and anus with soap and water, *before* sex. Take special care when washing the uncircumcised penis. The foreskin may trap germs.
- Use a condom, even if the woman is using a contraceptive.
- Use water based lubricants or jelly during intercourse so they wash away easily. Oil based lubricants such as petroleum jelly may leave a thin layer which will trap germs.
- Wash all around the genitals and anus *after* sex.
- Urinate immediately *before* and *after* sex. This helps wash the germs out of the urethra.

Douching the vagina is not a good idea, as it upsets the delicate skin and mucus of the vagina.

Prevent STDs by using a condom during intercourse.

The only sure way to avoid sexually transmitted diseases is to keep to one sexual partner. If everybody only had one partner, then STDs could not spread.

AIDS, or slim

AIDS stands for 'Acquired Immune Deficiency Syndrome'. This means that the body loses immunity to all diseases — whether common infections or rare cancers. AIDS is caught from other people, usually from sexual contact, through blood or semen. The disease can also be spread through infected injection needles or from **blood transfusions**. Most people who are infected will eventually develop AIDS and even if symptom free can still pass the disease on. Some others will develop less dangerous illnesses. AIDS *cannot* be caught from the air or from water or by shaking hands, touching, sharing cups or towels.

AIDS was only discovered in 1979,. AIDS is more common in Central Africa than other parts of Africa, though no-one knows why. Compared to many diseases AIDS is rare, but there is no known treatment. Scientists are working on a vaccine but it could take many years. Prevention is therefore the only cure. A few people carry AIDS in their blood for many years before the disease comes out. Most people die within three years of being diagnosed. They die from infections or rare cancers which cannot be treated.

The main groups of people at risk from AIDS are:
- Homosexual and bisexual men. AIDS is easily transferred by **anal** intercourse.
- People who have many sexual partners.
- Drug users who share injection needles.
- People who are given blood from unknown donors.
- Sexual partners of the above groups.
- Babies born to mothers with AIDS.

AIDS is very rare among anyone who is not in one of these groups.

The symptoms of AIDS are:
- Extreme tiredness lasting for several weeks with no obvious cause.
- Unexpected loss of weight of over 5 kg in two months.
- Fever, or night sweats lasting several weeks.
- Diarrhoea lasting several weeks.
- Painless flat hard lumps growing on the skin, or in the mouth or eyelids.
- Swollen glands, especially in the neck and armpits.
- Shortness of breath, gradually getting worse over several weeks, with a dry irritating cough.

All these symptoms occur with common diseases that are easily treated and are not AIDS. But if you fall into one of the high-risk groups and suffer from several of these symptoms then visit a clinic or hospital. Although there is no cure for AIDS, some of the infections can be treated. Tests can show if AIDS is in the blood.

Anyone who has AIDS, should *never* give blood, or parts of their body after their death. Alcohol and cigarettes should be avoided as they lower the body's resistance to infections. People with AIDS should *never* have sex with anyone, or they will infect their partners. AIDS is present in blood and semen and possibly in urine. If infected blood or semen gets into cuts in the skin it can infect that person. Toothbrushes and razors should not be shared with AIDS victims. There is no evidence that AIDS can be passed on through spit. Crockery and cutlery are quite safe if washed in hot water and detergent. There is no risk of catching AIDS in toilets, or swimming pools.

How to prevent AIDS:
- Do not have anal sex.
- Use a condom during sex.
- Keep to one sexual partner, or abstain from sex.

Which of these statements are true?

- You will know if you have got an STD.
- Only dirty people catch STDs.
- You cannot get an STD the first time you have sex.
- You catch gonorrhoea from toilet seats.
- You cannot get an STD more than once.
- You cannot have more than one STD at a time.
- Kissing spreads gonorrhoea.
- There is no cure for STDs.
- Once you have been treated, you cannot catch an STD again.
- An STD eventually goes away if you wait long enough.
- STDs are always the woman's fault.
- You have to have full sexual intercourse to catch an STD.
- If you have an STD you only have to tell your last partner.
- Sex with several partners one after the other will get rid of an STD.
- Having sex with a virgin will get rid of an STD.

None of these statements are true! They are *all* false.

Dear Auntie,

When I go to the toilet the urine is hot and burning. Five minutes later I want to go again, but there is nothing there. Could this be a sexually transmitted disease? I am a virgin, but I have heard you can catch diseases from toilet seats or washing towels.

Julia

Dear Julia,

Your symptoms are those of cystitis, infection of the bladder or urethritis, the tube leading from the bladder.

Because the urethra in a woman is very short, germs can easily get into the bladder. A virgin can catch this infection without sexual contact. Toilet seats or towels cannot give you a disease — the germs cannot live long enough. Not all infections of the female genitals are sexually transmitted.

A course of antibiotic tablets is the usual cure. See a health worker. Meanwhile drink as much water as you can, to help wash out the germs.

Dear Auntie,

My husband has returned after six months working in the city. He says I must go to the clinic for treatment for syphilis.

But I have no symptoms. I feel quite healthy, and I have never slept with anyone else. Why should I go when it is my husband who has been unfaithful to me? My mother has some traditional herbs which prevent and cure STDs. Shall I take these?

Mary

Dear Mary,

If your husband has caught syphilis while working in the city, then you must be treated too. Women can have a sexually transmitted disease without any symptoms, but the disease can still damage the body inside. If you are not treated soon then you will give the disease back to your husband.

The symptoms can take from a few days to some years before appearing. During all that time the disease is damaging the body inside.

There is no traditional treatment that will cure gonorrhoea or syphilis or any sexually transmitted diseases. You must be treated with modern antibiotic medicine at a clinic. Traditional medicines may stop the itching or pain, but they cannot cure the disease inside the body. You can still infect other people.

Dear Auntie,

I have some small sores on my penis. My cousin told me I should visit a Special Clinic, but I am afraid. A friend said he knew a man who went to such a clinic and the doctors wanted to cut off his penis. Can they really do this?

Peter

Dear Peter,

Friends like yours help the increase of sexually transmitted diseases by spreading wild and untrue rumours! No doctor would ever treat an STD by cutting off a man's penis. The treatment for all STDs is by medicines, either by swallowing tablets or by injection.

However small the sores are on your penis, you must visit the clinic. The health workers there will know how to treat you. No part of you will be cut!

If you are afraid or embarrassed, take your cousin with you to the clinic.

Activities

1 What are the most dangerous sexually transmitted diseases?

2 Discuss how the spread of STDs can be prevented.

3 Find out where the nearest clinic which treats STDs is. What times is it open? Discuss ways of encouraging people to attend STD clinics. Should treatment be free?

4 Draw a poster about preventing STDs.

5 Make up a role-play about a group of men who have different ideas about STDs and how to cure and prevent them. What happens to each man?

CHAPTER 7
Keeping clean and healthy

Keeping the body clean

Clean healthy skin helps the body to fight diseases. Try and wash the body all over every day. Skin sweats all the time but during exercise or hot weather it sweats more. Sweating helps the body to keep cool. The sweat evaporates and the body loses heat. Armpits sweat more than other parts of the body. Because the sweat cannot evaporate from the armpits it mixes with germs and starts to smell. A good wash with soap and warm water is usually enough to keep the body sweet-smelling.

A **deodorant** can help reduce the smell of stale sweat. Deodorants should not be used on top of old sweat — always wash it off first!

Some women feel more attractive if they shave their armpits.

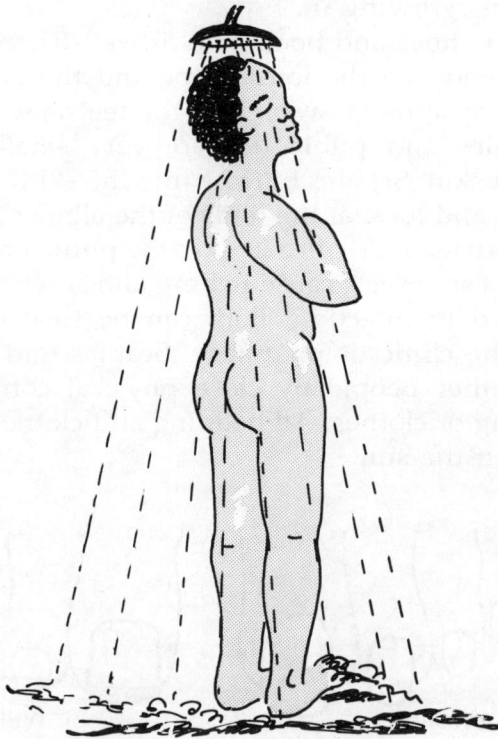

Showering.

This makes little difference to the smell. The skin of the armpits is very delicate so they must be careful not to cut or damage it.

Women should use mild soap on the genitals, not deodorants. Deodorants can cause irritation and soreness. They destroy the natural mucus and can cause infections of the vagina. Women should wipe their vulvas from front to back after using the toilet to prevent wiping germs from the anus into the vagina or urethra.

Everything you touch is covered in germs. Germs on your hands can get into food, either by touching the food, or by touching plates or cutlery. Germs in food can cause diarrhoea, vomiting and many other diseases.

Always wash the hands:
- Before preparing or eating food.
- After going to the toilet.
- When the hands look or feel dirty.

Sweaty feet smell bad and can develop skin infections.
- Wash the feet every day and dry them carefully between the toes.
- Wear clean socks or tights every day.
- Wear cotton or wool socks. Nylon fabrics make the feet sweat and smell more.
- Wear open sandals and no socks in hot weather.
- Keep the toe nails short. Cut them straight across to prevent the nails growing in.
- Wear shoes and boots that fit well. There should be one centimetre between the longest toe and the end of the shoes. Tight shoes cause more sweat and the feet may grow deformed.

Scabies and **pubic lice** are very small insects that live on human skin. Scabies burrow into the skin, especially between the fingers and toes, at the folds of the elbows and knees and around the genitals. Pubic lice live on the pubic hair around the genitals. Both these insects cause itching and soreness. Scratching the area can lead to infection. Both can be treated with special lotions from the clinic or pharmacy. Scabies and pubic lice are caught from other people by close physical contact, or from infested bedding or clothes. All bedding and clothes must be washed and dried in the sun.

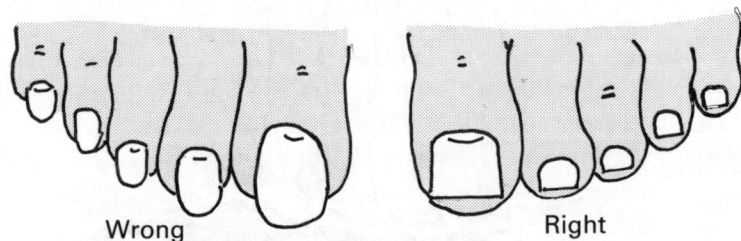

Wrong   Right

Cut toe nails straight across.

Teeth

Food and germs collect between teeth. This mixture of food and germs causes the gums to bleed and become inflamed. Gum disease does not hurt and many people think it is normal for their gums to bleed when they brush their teeth. They may stop brushing their teeth. But gum disease is caused by not brushing the teeth. The gums become red and swollen and the teeth appear longer. The teeth may become loose and eventually fall out.

Gum disease or rotten teeth can also cause bad breath and a bad taste in the mouth.

Brush your teeth before you go out on a date!

Food and germs cannot always be seen on or between the teeth. The only way to be sure that teeth are properly clean is to brush them twice a day for three minutes. Use a small toothbrush which reaches to the back of the mouth. A soft bristled toothbrush works better than hard bristles. Brush teeth up and down, not across, with small strokes so that the bristles get between the teeth. Clean the back teeth as thoroughly as the front teeth. Toothpaste does not help to get the germs and food out, but it does make the mouth taste nicer. Throw the toothbrush away when the bristles splay out. Or use a chewing stick. Chewing sticks made from local trees such as eucalyptus are as good as plastic toothbrushes.

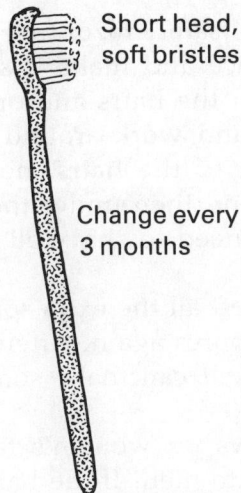

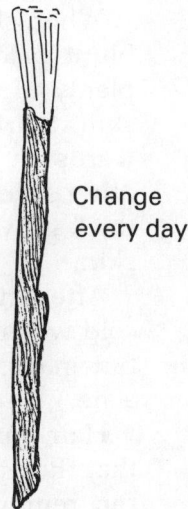

Short head, soft bristles

Change every 3 months

Change every day

Plastic toothbrush

Chewed stick brush

Different ways of cleaning teeth.

At first brushing the teeth twice a day for three minutes may make the gums bleed. Do not stop. Brushing away the dead food and germs will cure the bleeding and the gums will grow strong again.

Prevent gum disease by brushing teeth.

If you have a painful tooth visit a **dentist** who can fill the hole and prevent the tooth rotting further. The dentist may have to pull the whole tooth out to prevent the other teeth rotting.

Most people have all their main adult teeth by 16 years, with the four teeth at the back growing between 20 and 30 years.

Eating no sugar, sweets and fizzy drinks will prevent rotten teeth.

Hair

Greasy hair picks up dirt more easily than clean hair. Hair needs to be washed at least once a week, and more often in hot weather. Permed or bleached hair can become very dry. Try not to use so much oil that it drips onto other people or the backs of seats.

At puberty hair grows on a boy's face. First the hair grows on the upper lip, then on the cheeks and lastly on the lower chin. The first hair is soft and it gradually grows coarser. Whether to grow a beard or a moustache depends on fashion and local customs. If you want to shave, you do not have to wait until the hair is growing thickly.

When shaving with a 'safety razor' use a sharp, new blade. Old blunt blades cut the face and make it sore. Use hot water and plenty of soap to soften the hairs and open up the pores on the skin. Start at one ear and work around the chin. Shave downwards in the direction of the hairs, not against them. Do the other side of the face and then under the chin. If you have very thick growth you may need to shave all round again for smooth skin.

After shaving, wash off all the extra soap and then splash with cold water to close the pores again. Aftershave lotion smells nice, but may sting the face. It can make some skin dry and irritate acne.

Hair sometimes grows on women's faces. This is not a sign that they are turning into men! If the hair is very noticeable you can remove it with a special cream. Do not try to shave it as shaving will only make the hair grow thicker.

Clean bodies need clean clothes. Try to change underclothes and socks every day. Wash other clothes as soon as they are dirty.

Nylon fabrics need washing more often then natural fabrics like cotton and wool. But nylon fabrics are often cheaper, and they do not need ironing. Drying clothes in the sunshine helps to kill germs and make them smell fresh.

Acne

Acne is not a disease that can be caught from other people. Acne is caused by an imbalance of sex hormones at puberty. The hormones cause the natural skin oil to increase. The skin is covered in **sebaceous glands**, which produce natural oil. Some people have more oily skin than others.

New skin is constantly being made and old skin drops off. Acne spots are inflamed areas of skin, due to blocked skin pores. Pus may form and make an acne cyst.

Acne can be blackheads, oily skin with open skin pores or inflamed spots with pus.

Any part of the body with hairs can get acne. The face, shoulders, back and chest are most commonly affected.

Blackheads are spots with a black top. The black plug is a mixture of natural oils, dirt and skin, blocking the skin pore.

Most teenagers suffer from mild acne at some time. Greasy skin and occasional spots may last a few months, or come and go at random.

Severe acne is rare and usually affects young men. Acne occasionally affects children, or mature adults.

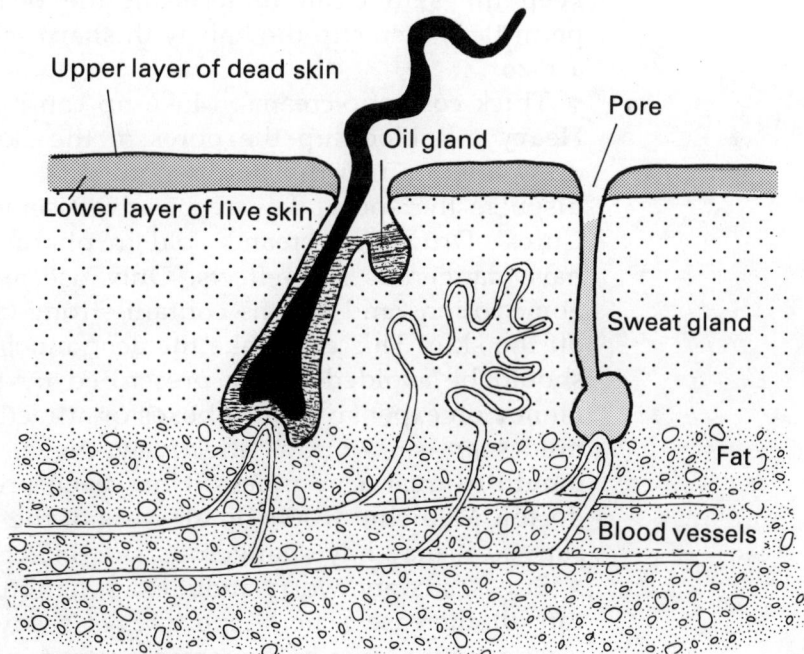

Inside the skin.

To help prevent acne avoid these

- Oil, grease or chemicals which irritate the skin. Wash all over with hot, soapy water immediately after work.
- Overalls soaked in machine oil or grease. Wear clean overalls every day.
- Working in hot, steamy kitchens. Keep the windows open. Do not stand for hours over greasy fumes from frying pans.
- Wearing nylon and man-made fabrics. Wear cotton and natural fibres, which absorb sweat and natural skin oil.
- Fluffy or rough wool, or harsh man made fabrics.
- Tight, stiff collars which rub the neck.
- Tight fitting denim jeans. These can cause acne on thighs and buttocks.
- The Pill. This can make acne worse for some women. Other women find their acne improves while taking the Pill. Many young women have spots a few days before a menstrual period. These clear up during or after the period.
- Hot smoky discos or bars. Go outside into the fresh air at intervals.
- Getting over tired and run down. Dancing and drinking do not directly affect acne. But too many late nights will reduce the body's resistance.
- Greasy hair held down by tight protective helmets or uniform hats. Hair oil encourages spots on the forehead. If the hairstyle needs oil, wear a scarf or ribbon around the hairline.

  Shaving may be very painful. Grow a beard, but remember to keep the skin clean underneath the beard. If a beard is not permitted, then clip the hair with sharp scissors rather than with a razor.
- Thick cosmetic creams. Make-up can make acne much worse. Heavy oils block up the pores of the skin. Shiny creams may draw attention to the bumps and pits on the skin, rather than disguise the spots. Beware of advertisements claiming 'Miracle Cures'. Drugs and creams sold in pharmacies to cure acne can have dangerous side-effects. Only use mild medicated creams. Some lotions and creams contain strong chemicals which 'burn' off the skin. This can make the acne much worse. Strong creams should be avoided unless prescribed by a clinic. Do not waste money on expensive fancy boxes or attractive bottles when cheap mild soap can work as effectively. Never take any medicine by mouth to treat acne unless it has been prescribed by a clinic or doctor. Medicine works on all parts of the body, and not just the skin so it may have dangerous side-effects.
- Stress, anxiety, worry about examinations, or problems at home can all increase acne. Acne always seems to get worse at the wrong time – just before an important interview, a special date or a party.

142

Treatment

Acne always clears up in the end — but it may take some years.

Spots and acne cannot be washed away, but skin should be kept clean to reduce the amount of oil and bacteria. Use mild, unperfumed soap. Antiseptic creams and transparent gels which kill bacteria and loosen blackheads should help mild acne.

Blackheads must only be squeezed with great care. Germs will make blackheads worse so wash the hands and face well with soap and hot water. Hot water softens the blackhead and skin. Do not squeeze with the fingernails as they bruise the skin. Never squeeze so hard that it hurts. If the blackhead does not come out, then leave it.

Fiddling, picking and squeezing spots only spreads them around the face and increases scarring. Some people scar more easily than others. Bad scars will eventually improve, but they may take some years.

Sunlight helps acne, though too much sweating increases acne.

No treatment works overnight. Be patient.

A healthy diet including plenty of fresh fruit and vegetables, and brown flour or rice will make the body healthier and able to overcome acne more effectively. Chocolate or fried foods encourage acne in some people. (See Keeping Healthy.)

Acne is not a disease that can be cured for ever. Some people have acne for years. They have to learn to live with it until they grow up.

Living with acne

Acne causes misery and discomfort and loss of self confidence to many young people. Worrying about acne may make it worse, and can affect the character. Personality is more important than good looks. Acne sufferers often feel lonely, but they are not the only sufferers — many of their friends will have it too. Most acne sufferers are so busy worrying about their own skin that they never notice anyone elses. Staying at home will not cure the acne, and will only increase the importance of the acne to you. Get out and enjoy yourself.

Sensitive people can become very disturbed by their acne, especially when their friends tease them with names like 'Spotty' or 'Scabby'. Ignoring such remarks is difficult, but it is the only way to stop them.

Many acne sufferers feel guilty. They believe the acne is their own fault, because of the way they think or behave. Neither sexual intercourse nor masturbation affects acne.

Acne occurs at just the age when young people are sensitive

143

about their looks and seeking friends and partners. Everyone wants the perfect film star face with a smooth glowing complexion. Many famous beautiful people have suffered from acne, or still do.

Severe acne should be treated by a clinic or doctor. Other skin conditions can look like acne, but need different treatment or have different causes.

Dear Auntie,

I am a 16 year old school boy and I wet my bed every night. I try not to drink in the afternoon, but still I wake up with wet blankets. I once tried traditional treatment, but it did no good. My problem is so embarrassing because even my friends at school complain about the smell.

Mohamed

Dear Mohamed,

This is more common than most bed wetters realise — many grown men wet their beds. There are several causes — infection of the bladder; weak bladder muscles; very deep sleep; stress or worry. Are you worrying a lot about school work? Your worry about your bed wetting may have become a vicious circle — the more you worry about it, the worse it becomes. Go to a clinic and ask for a **bilharzia** test. If that is negative then ask to be referred to a doctor who specialises in the urinary system.

Not drinking could cause other problems. Our bodies need lots of water to function and also to carry away waste products from the body. If you don't drink water, the bladder could be irritated and your urine will be stronger and smell more. Meanwhile, sleep with a plastic sheet and wash yourself and your clothes every morning.

Periods

If a woman does not wear something during her menstrual period then the menstrual blood will stain her clothes and trickle down her legs. This would be messy, uncomfortable and embarrassing.

A **sanitary towel** is a pad of cotton wool about 15 cm long, and 5 cm wide. Sanitary towels vary in size according to the amount of menstrual blood a woman has to cope with. Thinner more absorbent towels are a bit more expensive than thick larger towels.

Towels cover the vulva and absorb the blood as it leaves the vagina. Some towels are covered in fine cotton net with loops sewn on the ends. The loops are hooked on to an elastic belt worn around the waist. This type of cotton wool towel must be burnt, wrapped in paper or buried. Other towels are made from disposable material which can be flushed down a toilet. Never put a towel in a flush toilet unless the packet says on it 'Completely flushable or disposable'. Towels block up toilet pipes easily.

Some towels have sticky strips along the back. These are pressed onto the inside of the pants to hold the towel in place. These are comfortable, though they can become unstuck and crease up. They may have a plastic backing inside which prevents leaking.

'Mini-pads' or towels are smaller and thinner. They are not absorbent enough for the first days of a period. They are useful when a period is expected, or for the last couple of days when the flow is light. Or they can be worn for extra protection with a tampon.

Sanitary towels have to be changed every few hours, according to the menstrual flow. If left on too long they may begin to smell, or feel uncomfortable. Fresh menstrual blood does not smell until it has been in the air for a while. About four towels a day are needed, but every woman is different. Some women only bleed for three days, but their flow is heavy. Other women have a light period for eight days.

Some women put a handful of cotton wool in their pants. This is cheaper than towels, but not as absorbent. Bits of cloth can also be used but they are not so comfortable. Cloths can become infected if they are not washed properly and dried in the sun. To save money you can make washable sanitary towels (see instruction on page 146). Many women are embarrassed to hang their

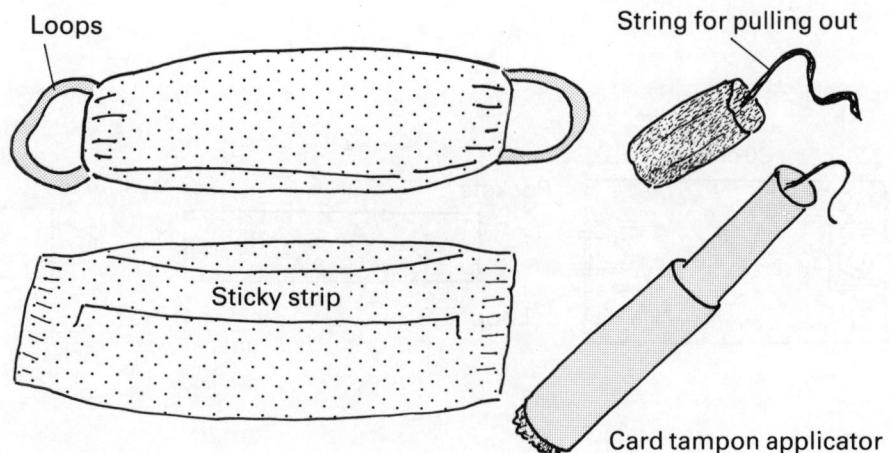

Loops

String for pulling out

Sticky strip

Card tampon applicator

Sanitary towels and tampons.

sanitary cloths outside to dry. If cloths are dried inside they can grow mould and this can lead to vaginal infections. Fresh air and sunshine are important for killing germs. At the end of each period all the cloths should be boiled and then kept in a clean dry place for next time. Use flowered or patterned fabric so that stains do not show.

Close fitting pants are needed to hold all types of sanitary towels in place.

To make washable sanitary towels

90 cm × 100 cm will make 12 towels. The fabric must be cotton — man made or nylon fabrics are not absorbent and cannot be boiled.

Materials needed

To make one towel
One piece of coloured cotton 30 cm × 15 cm
Two small pieces of cloth 5 cm × 5 cm
Two strips of cloth 10 cm × 2 cm, or two tapes 10 cm long

Instructions

1 Sew the two small pieces of cloth onto the ends of the main piece like pockets. At the same time sew the ends of the narrow strips, or tapes in between the large piece and the pockets to form a loop.
2 Fold the sides of the cloth back to make a long thin rectangle.
3 Turn the two pockets inside out, pulling the loops out. Wear folded like this. For a heavy flow, put cotton wool or kapok inside the folded cloth. Unfold to wash and dry. No-one will know these are sanitary towels. To make them last longer sew a hem around the edges of the cloth.

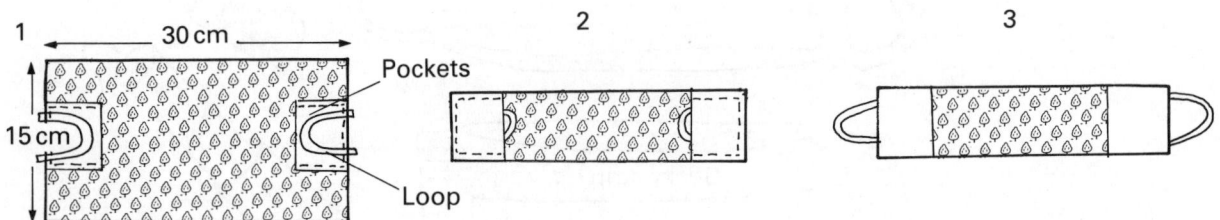

How to make a washable sanitary towel.

Tampons

A **tampon** is a tight roll of cotton wool placed inside the vagina to absorb the menstrual blood as it leaves the uterus. Each tampon is about 4 cm long and 1 cm across with 10 cm of string at one end. Some tampons are inserted with a finger. Others are sold with a special applicator made from two tubes of cardboard which are thrown away after use. The string remains outside the vagina to pull out the used tampon. The muscles of the vagina hold the tampon in place. Tampons cannot get lost inside a woman. The hole at the top of the vagina is no bigger than a pin. If the string is pushed up inside the vagina it can easily be reached with the fingers by squatting with the knees bent.

The advantage of tampons is that they cannot be felt or seen, even if very tight trousers are worn. With tampons a woman can take part in every type of sport − even swimming. She can forget that she is having a period.

Most girls can use tampons from their first period. Very few women cannot use tampons, it just takes patience and practice. Every packet is sold with instructions and if these are followed carefully then learning to use tampons is easy.

Remember to relax all the muscles and to take your time. If the tampon can be felt, then it is not inserted correctly. Try again with another one. The vagina does not go straight up from the vulva. It slants towards the back. Before trying to insert a tampon for the first time, feel with the fingers the angle of the vagina. If the hymen is too tight, then try again in a few months.

Tampons are sold in different sizes, according to a woman's size and how much she bleeds. There are small tampons for young unmarried women and larger sizes for women with heavy periods or who have had babies.

Tampons usually need changing about every four hours − more often than towels. They cannot be seen so it is more difficult to know when they need changing. When the tampon is full, the string will be stained. At night a tampon is not always enough, so wear a mini-pad or towel as well. On a long journey when changing tampons or towels is difficult, two tampons can be inserted together. This is not advisable as a normal habit, but only for emergencies.

Always remember to take out the last tampon at the end of a period. Tampons are so comfortable that it is easy to forget. If a tampon is left in by mistake it can cause infection, fever or serious illness. Remember to take out the used tampon before inserting a new one each time.

Try out all the different methods of sanitary wear to find out which suits you best. Always carry a tampon or towel in your bag so that you are not caught out when your period starts. If your period starts unexpectedly, then put some rolled up tissues or a clean handkerchief in your pants until you can get home or go to a shop.

Washing stained pants or cloths

Hot water will 'cook' blood into fabric. Soak blood stains in cold water with a little salt added. Fresh blood washes out easily in cold soapy water. If the blood has dried, then it may need a few hours soaking.

Dear Auntie,

I am a guy of 20 who is too embarrassed to go swimming or bathe in front of others because I have a bulging navel. Is there anything that can be done?

Washington

Dear Washington,

A bulging navel, or umbilical hernia is fairly common among both men and women. It is caused by a gap in the muscles of the abdomen which hold in the intestines. An umbilical hernia is not dangerous, but can be treated with a small operation by sewing the muscles together. Hernias on other parts of the abdomen or groin can be dangerous as they may pinch the intestines and cut off the blood supply.

If you try not to be self-conscious about your hernia then people will not notice. No body is 100% perfect!

Food

Adolescents grow very fast — both in height and weight — so they need to eat plenty of good food. Even when the body is fully grown eating well is important to keep healthy. Good food is needed for energy, to fight off diseases, and to repair the body.

A healthy diet consists of a mixture of all types of food. Eat some food from each of these groups every day.

- Growing foods:
Nuts, eggs, beans, meat, fish, milk, cheese, insects.
- Energy foods:
Maize, cassava, plantain, bread, rice, potatoes, margarine.
- Protective foods:
Fresh fruit, vegetables, eggs, margarine, milk.

The body needs **fibre** to prevent constipation and reduce the risk of digestive diseases. Fibre is found in brown bread and rice, unrefined flour and maize, fruit, vegetables, beans and nuts.

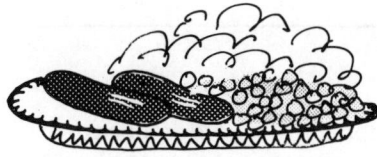

Maize, meat and green cabbage

Rice, eggs and carrots and orange

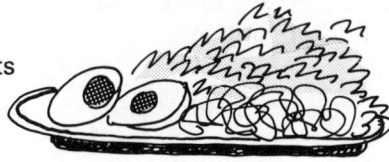

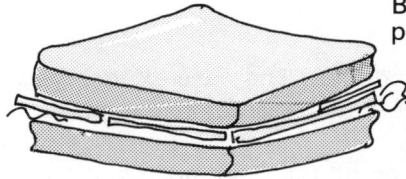

Brown bread, margarine, peanut butter and mango

Balanced meals.

Fibre fills up the stomach, without being fattening or giving energy. Foods such as white bread or rice, refined maize meal, milk, cooking oil and sweets do not contain fibre.

Foods fried in oil or fat are not as healthy as boiled, baked or steamed foods. They are also more fattening and may encourage spots.

Many foods taste good, but do not help the body. Some foods, such as herbs, spices, tea and coffee do no harm in small quantities. Salt is needed in very small amounts. Most people eat far too much salt on their food. Too much salt overworks the kidneys of babies and children. In adults salt can cause high blood pressure, which is especially dangerous in pregnant women. Foods such as potato crisps, bread, ready cooked meats and tinned food have salt already added. Meat, eggs and milk contain natural salt.

Sweet, fizzy, cool drinks are an expensive way of drinking coloured, sweetened water with bubbles of air. Fizzy drinks, sweets and sugar rot the teeth. Peanuts, a boiled egg, fruit or bread and margarine make better snacks than sweets.

Advertisements of prepared food make them look very delicious, but they are more expensive and less good for you. Ready made foods often contain chemicals to give the food colour and taste. Some of these chemicals can harm the body. Fresh food is healthier, cheaper and contains no added chemicals. Avoid eating too many tinned, dried, packet or prepared foods.

Eat more fresh food for a healthy body.

149

Dear Auntie,

I am a girl of 20 years but I look much older because I am so fat. My shoulders are not too bad, but my bottom is very big. Would slimming pills help my problem?

Marie

Dear Marie,

Slimming pills are not a good idea. They are expensive and you can become addicted to them and so cause much greater problems. In many countries they are illegal.

First, stop worrying about being fat. The more you worry the more you will feel hungry and the more you will then eat. All women have bigger bottoms than men. Women are designed for having babies — they have wide hips so that the baby can be born easily. They also store fat in their bottoms and legs in case of famine.

If you weigh more than in the chart then adjust your eating habits. Do not go on a 'crash' diet hoping to eat nothing for a week. This never works and can be dangerous as you must eat some food. To lose weight eat lots of fresh fruit and vegetables and drink only water. Drink lots of water before meals, to make you feel full. You can eat as much bread, maize, rice, cassava or yams as you like. But only with fresh, boiled or raw vegetables. Fatty meat, fried foods and cooking oil will make you fat. Jam, margarine, butter, sugar, cool drinks and alcohol are out too. Chew your food slowly, so that it takes longer to eat. Don't eat sweets, biscuits, cakes, puddings or fried foods. Fresh fruit and vegetables will help you get slim. Accept yourself as a woman, but reduce your weight to the right one for your height.

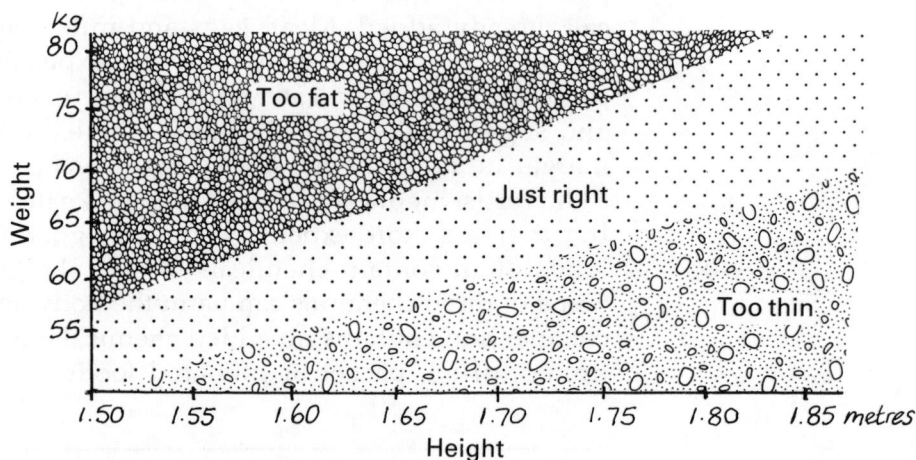

Recommended weight for height chart.

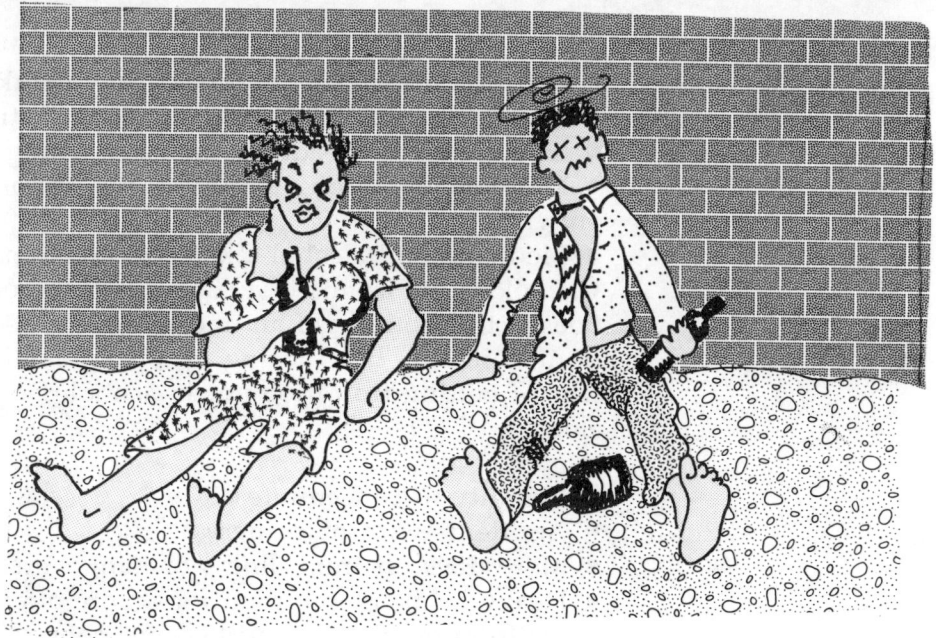

Getting drunk does not make anyone tall, rich, strong, handsome, beautiful, clever, smart or sexy.

Alcohol

Many religions ban the drinking of alcohol. This is because alcohol can damage people. It is bad for their health, their work and their families.

Alcohol makes some people feel friendly and amusing while other people feel quiet and depressed. Drinking alcohol can be an enjoyable way to relax with friends. If you drink too much, or at the wrong time, you will make problems. Alcohol affects all parts of the body. It is a depressant, which slows down the body and brain. Every time you drink alcohol, it affects your judgement, self control and skill; thinking and re-acting take longer. If you drink a lot of alcohol for several years, it will damage the body and brain.

Problems that occur from alcohol

Health
- Damage to nervous system, heart and brain.
- Serious damage to liver, or kidneys.
- Stomach ulcers.
- Depression.
- Reduced immunity to disease.
- Wounds and sores heal more slowly.
- Alcohol prevents blood from clotting, so bleeding is heavier after accidents. **Never** give alcohol to someone after an accident — it slows down the heart and encourages bleeding.
- Vitamin deficiency because alcohol absorbs essential vitamins.
- Malnutrition. Heavy drinkers replace food with alcohol. Alcohol

151

is not food, though it can give heavy drinkers fat stomachs.
- Blindness or death from homemade distilled alcohol.
- 'Hangovers' — headache, nausea, aching body.
- Pregnancy — alcohol goes into the unborn baby and slows its growth.
- Medicine and alcohol taken together can be very dangerous.
- Choking on vomit is a common cause of death from alcohol. Loosen the clothing of an unconscious person. Lie them on their front, with the head facing to one side. Vomiting is the body's way of getting rid of too much alcohol. Do not leave this person alone.

Work
- Inability to concentrate.
- Accidents with machinery.
- More days off from illness or hangovers.
- Heavy drinkers lose their jobs more often. They get bad references from employers and become poor.

Home
- A parent who has drunk too much alcohol may hit a child. The parents may not care for the children properly.
- Arguments or fights between friends and relations.
- Alcohol costs a lot of money, so there is less money for family needs, such as food.
- Sexual difficulties. After drinking men feel sexually aroused. They may try to rape their wives or other women. But sometimes drunk men cannot have an erection.
- Women may forget about the risks of pregnancy, or catching an STD. They may say 'Yes' to a man, when they do not really mean it.
- Men may forget about their responsibilities to their wives and families.
- Road accidents which kill or injure drivers, passengers and pedestrians. A motorist makes almost twice as many mistakes after just one bottle of beer. Moving the eyes to look for danger takes one fifth longer. But because alcohol makes people feel good, they believe that they are driving even better than usual!

In a test professional drivers drank alcohol and then drove between some posts. The more they had to drink the more confident they were that they could do it — and the more posts they knocked over!

Drinking and driving does not only affect the drinker — it can kill or injure innocent passengers and pedestrians. Road accidents after drinking are the main cause of death in young men.

Do not drink and drive.

- Alcohol is especially dangerous when using machinery at work.
- Alcohol reduces willpower. Drinking can easily become a habit which is very hard to stop.

How much is too much?

- Alcohol affects people in different ways according to their height, weight, sex and how much they have eaten before they drink.
- Women are more affected by alcohol than men because men's bodies contain more water. So the alcohol becomes more diluted in men. Also most men are larger than most women.
- Any man of average size will suffer from illness related to alcohol if he drinks 4 pint bottles of beer a day or more.
- Any woman of average size will suffer from alcohol related illness if she drinks 2½ bottles of beer a day, or more.
- 'Extra strength' lagers are three times as strong as ordinary beer.
- Mixing spirits with soft drinks can be dangerous. The taste of the alcohol is hidden by the sweet soft drinks. A man can drink a whole bottle of brandy without realising it — until he falls to the floor!

Many people with drinking problems are not aware of how much they drink every day. They believe that they only drink a small amount, when they are really drinking enough to harm their health, or affect their work. If you are drinking more than four bottles of beer a day, or its equivalent then you should think about reducing the amount you drink.

- Do not keep alcohol in the home.
- Choose tea, coffee or soft drinks more often.
- Drink water or fruit squash to quench your thirst, not beer.
- Drink small bottles of beer, rather than large ones.

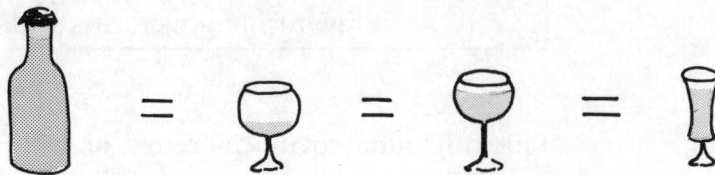

All these contain the same amount of alcohol.
Small bottle of beer or lager — small measure of spirits — glass of wine — small glass of sherry.

- Keep a count of each drink with matchsticks or coins.
- Give yourself rewards for drinking less — like a delicious meal or an outing.
- Keep an account of the money you save by drinking less.
- Change your social habits. Think about where you drink the most and avoid visiting those places.
- If you go to a bar every night, go there later each evening. Do not plan to leave early — you will not manage it!
- Eat a large meal before going out. A plate of food or a pint of milk before drinking absorbs some of the alcohol.
- Talk about your problem with a friend or relation.
- Never drink home distilled alcoholic spirits.

Hangovers

A hangover is the body's reaction to alcohol, which is a mild poison.

Many people wake up after a night of drinking feeling terrible. They have a bad headache and nausea, their limbs ache and they cannot think straight. There are many 'Special Cures' for hangovers — some of them even contain more alcohol! No hangover is cured by drinking more. Some of the symptoms are helped by aspirin or paracetamol.

Dehydration, or lack of water in the body is one effect of drinking too much. Drink as much water, tea or fruit squash as possible.

There is no fast way of making the effect of alcohol wear off. One small measure of whisky takes one hour to wear off. One pint of whisky or four pints of beer will take eight hours to wear off. After a heavy night of drinking a man can wake up in the morning still drunk.

Some alcohol causes worse hangovers because it contains added poisonous ingredients, such as colouring or flavouring. Homemade alcohol is the most dangerous of all. It may be very strong and can cause blindness or death.

Prevent hangovers — drink less alcohol.

Smoking

Smoking tobacco in cigarettes or a pipe is a habit enjoyed by many people. All of these people are harming their health.

Why is smoking bad for you?

- Smoking ruins your health. Most heavy smokers die from diseases caused by smoking. Tobacco contains poisonous **tar, nicotine** and **carbon monoxide**. Nicotine makes the heart beat faster and narrows the blood vessels. This contributes to heart and blood circulation diseases, both major causes of death among smokers. Exhaust fumes from motor cars also contain carbon monoxide. Would you put your mouth to an exhaust pipe of a car?

• Smoking makes you cough. The tar in tobacco sticks to the delicate passages in the lungs. Dirt, bacteria and mucus are trapped in the lungs. The lungs become inflamed, causing the 'smoker's cough'. Bronchitis and pneumonia are common among smokers.

The only safe cigarette is an unlit one.

• Most people who die of lung cancer have smoked tobacco. There is no cure for lung cancer. Cancer slowly and painfully grows to block the lungs. Other types of cancer are also more common in smokers. 'Low tar' cigarettes are just as dangerous.

• Smoking leads to mouth infections and stomach ulcers. Nicotine is absorbed into the blood and irritates the stomach lining.

• Smoking lowers the resistance to many diseases. Smokers catch diseases like 'flu more often.

• Every cigarette shortens your life by 14 minutes. Giving up smoking *now* will make you live longer and be healthier.

It is never too late to give up smoking.

• Days are lost at work or school through smoking illness. This costs you money, and holds back your education.

• Smokers get out of breath and tired quickly. They never make good sportsmen or sportswomen. The lungs become lined with tar. The more a person smokes, the more tar will be in their lungs. Smokers always puff and pant when they run. The blood vessels become narrower, so that blood cannot flow through them as quickly. Some smokers have to have their legs cut off because the blood vessels are blocked from smoking.

Successful sportsmen never smoke.

• Smoking spoils the sense of taste and smell. Smokers cannot enjoy their food and drink as much as non-smokers.

• Smoking spoils the appetite for food.

• Smoking makes hair, clothes and breath smell of stale smoke. Who wants to smell like yesterday's ashtray? Non-smokers never enjoy being close to smokers.

Kiss a non-smoker and taste the difference.

- Smoking stains teeth and fingers an unattractive colour. Imagine the black colour of a smoker's lungs.
- Smoking is expensive. The money could be used to improve your health, or life style, rather than ruining it. How many cigarettes cost the same as a record, or a pair of shoes?

The car of your dreams is in your ashtray.

Why is smoking bad for others?

- Other people have to breathe in the smoke from your cigarettes. Babies' and children's delicate lungs may be damaged if they breathe in your cigarette smoke.
- Children of smokers are more likely to become smokers themselves.
- Pregnant women who smoke harm their unborn babies. The baby grows slower and may be born smaller and weaker.
- Breastfeeding mothers who smoke have nicotine in their milk.
- Other people have to smell your smoky clothes, hair and breath.
- Other people have to look at your yellow teeth.
- Smokers take up valuable time with doctors and clinics. Health workers are busy enough with diseases that cannot be avoided.
- Smokers take more days off from work. This costs you, your family and your country money.
- Tobacco is grown on land that could be growing food crops.

Why do people like smoking?

- Smoking makes them feel adult. But being adult means being responsible for one's body and health − not trying to destroy it.
- Smoking makes them feel clever. But clever people know the damage smoking does to their health.
- Because all their friends smoke. But why kill yourself just because your friends want to die?
- They like the feeling of giving and receiving cigarettes with their friends. Try sharing nuts or fruit instead.
- Smoking gives them something to do with their hands. Try knitting, sewing, playing cards, or tying knots in a piece of string instead. Put your hands in your pockets.
- It gives them something to suck. Try chewing gum, eating fruit or sucking a smooth stone.
- It gives them a jumpy feeling of energy. Nicotine gives the body short bursts of energy. If you are tired, eat something or sit down for a rest.

The sooner you stop smoking, the better for your health.

How to stop smoking

● Remember that every cigarette is poisoning your body. The human body was not designed to smoke. You do not smoke while asleep, so why smoke while awake?

● It is not easy to stop smoking, especially if it has become a habit for a long time. Making the decision to stop is half the battle. Take it one day at a time. Each day that you do not smoke is an achievement.

● Plan a day to stop on. From that day you are not a 'Smoker trying to stop' — you are a Non-Smoker. On that day throw away everything to do with cigarettes — lighters, ashtrays, and half packets of cigarettes.

● Persuade a friend, relation, husband or wife to stop too. Giving up is easier if you support each other. If a pregnant woman and her husband stop smoking together they will improve the health of three people at once!

● Work out where and when you smoke most. Plan ways of avoiding these times. If you always smoke after a meal, get up straight away and do something else.

● Tell all your friends that you have stopped, then it will be more difficult to go back on your word. Ignore them if they joke and try and tempt you to start again. Make a bet with someone that you *can* stop smoking.

● Every time you want a cigarette breathe deeply and listen to your breathing. Think about your lungs becoming blocked up with tar. Breathing slowly will make you feel calm.

● Work out how much money you are saving by not smoking. Put it aside to buy something special for yourself or your family. Imagine that every cigarette you smoke is a rolled up note of money.

Why pay to kill yourself?

● Think of all the advantages of not smoking. You smell fresher, you breathe clean air, you have more money, you are less likely to die young, you are more attractive, and you can prove to yourself that you can control your life.

● Learn to play a musical instrument that needs blowing, such as a trumpet. Take up a sport like football. Notice the difference — now you can run.

● At the end of the first day, or week, give yourself a treat — something nice to eat, or a trip to the cinema.

● Gather together some friends to start a group of people giving

157

up smoking. Meet once a week and discuss how to give up. Those who have given up can help those who are about to. Discuss your successes and failures.

● Do not be tempted by 'Just one cigarette' — the odd one can lead to another, and another. Remember that you are now a Non-Smoker.

> Always say 'No' to cigarettes.

Heavy smokers may get irritable or lack concentration for the first days or even weeks of not smoking. Ask your family to be patient with you — a few bad days are better than dying early. Your cough may get worse at first as the lungs clean themselves out.

People often put on weight when they give up smoking because their appetite has returned and food tastes better. Eat more fresh fruit and vegetables and less fatty or sweet foods. (See Keeping Healthy page 148.) Do not use putting on weight as an excuse to return to smoking.

If you cannot give up all at once, then cut down the amount you smoke. Only smoke half a cigarette. Start smoking an hour later each day. Cut out one cigarette every day until you smoke none at all.

Many people have to try a few times before they stop smoking for ever. In Britain alone, eight million people have managed to give up smoking.

> Out of 1,000 young men who smoke, 250 will die early because of tobacco.

Smoking myths

Myth: 'Smoking kills germs in the lungs and prevents colds.'
Truth: The only thing that smoking will kill is *you*.

___

Myth: 'One or two every now and then will not do any harm.'
Truth: '*Every* cigarette is 14 minutes off your life.'

___

Myth: 'It is my life to do what I want with, so why shouldn't I smoke?'
Truth: You may be influencing children into a dangerous habit. And your sickness or early death will affect those you love around you.

___

Myth: 'Doctors smoke so it must be OK.'
Truth: More doctors have given up smoking than any other profession.

___

Drugs

All drugs and medicines can be dangerous, but only some are illegal. In most countries buying, selling, using or growing **cannabis, heroin, cocaine** and **LSD** is illegal. Allowing someone else to use one's property to keep or use drugs is also illegal. In some countries drug dealers are executed or receive long prison sentences. Arrest, prosecution and conviction affects the drug user's education and career, even if they are not sent to prison. Drug abuse damages health and causes social, mental, and legal problems to the user and the community. Operating machinery and using roads become very dangerous for both the drug user and others.

Buying drugs in the streets or from friends is illegal and dangerous. Always refuse any pills, powders or strange cigarettes.

Always say 'No' to drugs.

Drug users need larger and larger amounts of the drug to satisfy them. **Addiction**, or dependence occurs when a person cannot live without drugs. They will do anything to get hold of the drug. They might steal, break into drug stores, or even murder. Physical addiction makes the body react painfully when the drug is stopped. Mental dependence means that a person believes they cannot live without the drug. Treatment for addiction and dependence is possible, but it takes time and patience.

Pregnant women who use drugs affect both themselves and the unborn baby. The baby may be born addicted, or die around the time of birth. Some drugs can cause a miscarriage or make the baby deformed.

Injecting drugs is the most dangerous way to take them. An injected drug goes straight into the blood stream and reaches the brain within seconds.

Dangers of injecting drugs

- **Overdose** — a small amount of injected drug has a stronger effect on the body.
- Infections such as **hepatitis** and AIDS are spread by sharing injection needles.
- Gangrene (rotting flesh) can be caused by injecting the wrong blood vessel.
- Blood poisoning can be caused by dirty needles or dirty water.
- Infections can be caused by injecting crushed tablets.
- Addiction is more common when drugs are injected, because larger doses are used.

Addiction takes time. So anyone taking drugs should give up

now, before addiction develops. Mixing drugs is very dangerous. Small amounts of two drugs can cause fatal overdoses.

Why do people use drugs?

- Curiosity.
- They want to try something forbidden by their parents.
- They want to try something illegal.
- Boredom.
- To escape from problems.
- Seeking thrills and excitement.
- Influenced by friends.

The effects of drugs vary according to:

- The amount taken. Too much at once can cause accidents, or death.
- The size of the person. Small, light people are in more danger from overdose of drugs.
- How often they are taken. Taking drugs frequently can lead to addiction, or damage the body. The cost of expensive drugs leads to poor diet, bad housing, disease or stealing for money and imprisonment.
- The health of the user. Someone already suffering from mental illness may be badly affected by drugs. Some drugs reduce resistance to disease. Others directly affect parts of the body.
- The strength of the drug, which may not be known. Illegal drugs are often mixed with sugar, talcum powder or flour to make more profit for the dealer. A drug user never knows the strength of the drug.

Alcohol, barbiturates, opium, heroin and morphine are all **depressants**, which slow down the brain and the heart rate. There is less ability to control social behaviour, which results in accidents, violence, or promiscuity. Depressant drugs can make people feel aggressive, because inhibitions are weakened.

Miraa, amphetamines, and cocaine are **stimulants** which increase mental activity and heart rate. Stimulants give a false feeling of energy and well being. Sleep is not needed, but after a few days the body reacts by collapsing. Convulsions and mental illness can occur.

Cannabis and LSD cause hallucinations which are like bad dreams, while awake. The person imagines things that are not really there and may become very frightened.

Heroin, (or horse, smack, Big H.)

Heroin is a white powder made from the opium poppy, which is swallowed, smoked, inhaled or mixed with water and injected.

Heroin is the most expensive of all drugs so is often connected with corruption, crime and gangsters. The high cost of heroin leads to stealing.

Short term effects	Heroin relieves pain. It reduces brain activity, coughing, breathing and the heart rate. There is a feeling of calmness and warmth. Problems are forgotten. It may cause vomiting or constipation.
Long term effects	Addiction will occur. The user needs heroin just to feel normal. A heroin addict who stops taking heroin, will suffer from aching body, diarrhoea, vomiting, sweating, and muscular spasms which may last seven to ten days. There will be weakness for several months. Damage to the body is also caused by dirty injection needles, dirty water, reduced appetite leading to poor diet and lowered immunity to disease.
Cocaine, (or snow, coke)	Cocaine is a very expensive white powder made from the leaves of a South American bush. Cocaine is smoked or sniffed up the nose.
Short term effects	Excitement, mental stimulation and reduced hunger occur. It relieves pain and tiredness. There is a feeling of great strength; also sometimes anxiety, and panic. The effect lasts for about 30 minutes. Large doses may cause anxiety, hallucinations and death from breathing failure or heart attack.
Long term effects	The after effect of tiredness and depression leads users to take more cocaine. They may want to return to the feeling of well-being. Happiness is replaced by restlessness, excitablity, sickness, sleeplessness and weight loss. Regular users become nervous, suspicious and confused due to lack of sleep. Sniffing cocaine damages the inside of the nose.
Sniffing	The fumes from glue, nail varnish, paint, aerosol gas and petrol are inhaled, sometimes from inside a plastic bag.
Short term effects	This is similar to strong alcohol, only more dangerous. The person's breathing and heart rate slow down. There is a general loss of control, with a feeling of being in a dream. Sometimes the user falls unconscious. After half an hour the person suffers from headaches, vomiting and poor concentration. After a lot of sniffing the user becomes tired, forgetful and depressed with lack of concentration, and loss of weight. Accidental injury or death can occur from loss of control, choking on vomit if unconscious, or suffocation from putting plastic bags over the head or squirting gas into the mouth.

| Long term effects | The chemicals damage the brain, kidneys, liver, bones, lungs and lining of the nose. |

Amphetamines, (sulphate or speed)

Amphetamine tablets are made for medical use for relieving depression and sleepiness. Illegal drug dealers sell them for a feeling of energy, confidence and happiness. These effects wear off after a few hours, leaving the person feeling tired, anxious, and restless. High doses cause panic, hallucinations, or fear of persecution. To maintain the 'speedy' effects users have to increase the dose. When they finally stop they feel depressed, dull, and very hungry. Amphetamines are addictive.

Tranquillizers (or hypnosedatives, barbiturates)

Tranquillizers are used by doctors to calm excited people down and to help them to sleep. Tranquillizers are similar to alcohol, but stronger. They too are addictive. Large doses cause unconsciousness, breathing difficulties, and death. If mixed with alcohol, sedatives are even more dangerous and may kill. They can also cause bronchitis and pneumonia.

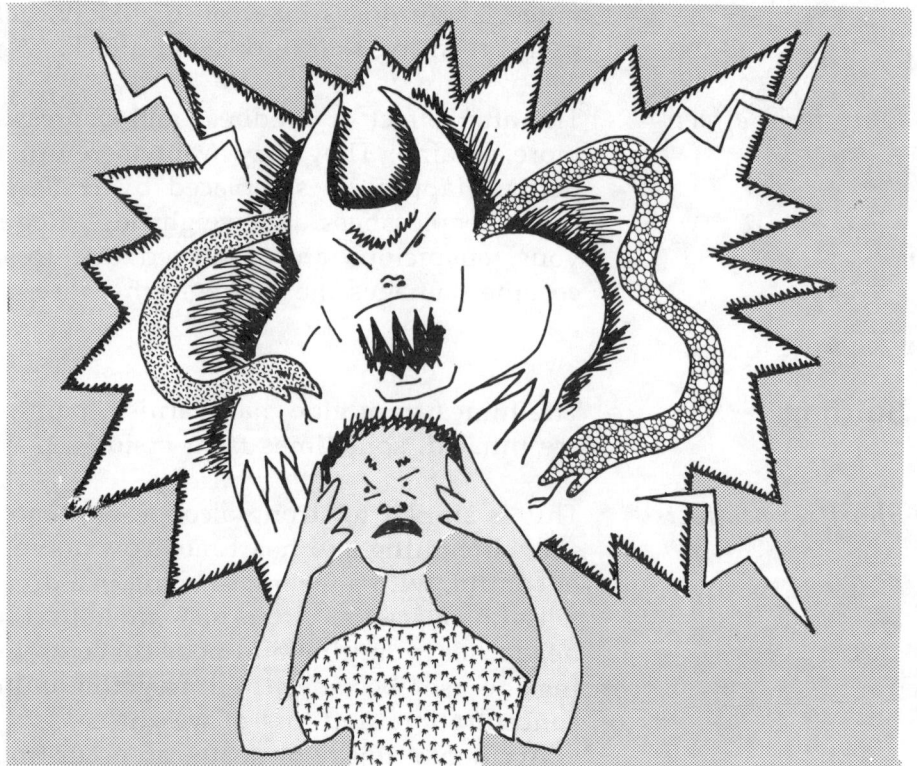

Hallucinations can be very frightening.

A tranquillizer addict who stops using tranquillizers will suffer from irritability, nervousness, sickness, twitching, convulsions or brain damage. Stopping their use suddenly can kill.

Cannabis

Cannabis is also known as bhang, dope, dhagga, grass, marijuana, hashish or ganja. It is the leaves or pollen of a plant, which is smoked in pipes or mixed with tobacco in cigarettes.

Short term effects

Users feel relaxed, and forget their worries. They enjoy sounds and colours more. Moods are increased, so depressed users become more depressed, and happy users become happier. Higher doses can cause panic, depression, or hallucinations. Driving or using machinery is dangerous after using cannabis. Normally there is no hangover.

Long term effects

The smoke from cannabis can cause bronchitis and breathing problems. Frequent users of cannabis may appear dull, and neglect their health and appearance and care less for their family and children. Memory and concentration are affected.

People with existing heart, lung, breathing or mental problems are at increased risk from cannabis.

Drug dealers often begin by selling young people cannabis. When the dealer knows the young person is dependent on cannabis, stronger and more dangerous drugs, such as heroin, are offered − perhaps free the first time. Hard drugs, such as heroin and cocaine, are the really dangerous ones − and where the big profits are made by drug dealers.

LSD, (or acid)

LSD is a strong chemical which is swallowed in tablets, on sugar cubes or soft paper. The strength of each dose is always unknown and the effect cannot be predicted. LSD affects the mind and not the body. A large dose of LSD can drive a person mad. Some people feel calm, peaceful and forget about time. Other people panic, and have hallucinations. 'Bad trips' may include depression, dizziness, or terror of imagined things. These feelings last about a day but some people behave strangely for many months. Some people think that nothing can harm them, so they walk in front of cars, or jump off buildings.

Miraa

Miraa is a green stick that is chewed. It is a stimulant that makes the user stay awake for long periods and lose the appetite. Although legal in some countries miraa is not good for the health. It causes stomach ulcers, rotten teeth, and accidents due to lack of concentration. The after-effects of chewing miraa for some hours are tiredness, depression and hunger.

Herbs and mushrooms

There are many different varieties of herbs or mushrooms that if eaten or smoked have powerful effects similar to LSD. Users may have hallucinations and stomach pains, or they may vomit. The effect may last several days. Many of these 'natural drugs' are poisonous and can kill the user if too much is used at once. The greatest danger is eating a fatally poisonous mushroom or herb by mistake. Identification can be very difficult.

How to give up drugs

There is only one person who can help a user to give up drugs. That person is the user. Until the user decides that he or she wants to stop using dangerous drugs, other people cannot help.

Some drugs are easier to give up than others. Addictive drugs, such as heroin and tranquillizers can cause painful or unpleasant withdrawal symptoms, which may be difficult to cope with.

- Make a decision to give up using drugs. Keep to your plan.
- Get advice and help from a doctor who will support you. Most doctors will not tell the police if you go to them for help in confidence. Often churches will help people to give up drugs.
- Work out why you use drugs. Plan to improve your life so that you do not need drugs.
- Work out where you use drugs. Plan to avoid the people and places where temptation is greatest. If possible, move away from the area for a few weeks.
- Ask a friend to give up with you. Or get support from a friend who does not use drugs, but will help you.
- Plan new activities to use the time you have used with drugs.
- Plan how to reduce your drug use, or stop altogether. Some drugs such as cannabis, can be given up immediately. Others, such as heroin may need reducing slowly over a few days or weeks. Giving up suddenly may result in bad withdrawal effects which send you back onto drugs. Stopping barbiturates suddenly can be dangerous.
- Remember that every day away from drugs will keep you healthier, and safe from prosecution.

Activities

1 Discuss the advantages of keeping clean.
2 What foods are good for you? Cook or plan some balanced meals.
3 Draw a poster about the dangers of tobacco, or alcohol, or drugs.

4   Make up a role-play about a teenager who becomes addicted to drugs or alcohol. How does it start? What happens in the end?
5   Discuss ways of preventing the abuse of alcohol, drugs or tobacco.
6   If you smoke cigarettes, stop smoking THIS week, not next month.
7   If you know anyone who uses illegal drugs tell them about the dangers to their health.

Glossary

Abdomen	the area of the body between the chest and legs.
Abortion	[a-BOR-shn] operation to remove a foetus from the uterus, usually through the vagina.
Abstinence	not having sexual intercourse.
Abscess	[AB-sis] a sac of pus caused by infection.
Acne	[AK-nee] spots on face, neck or back.
Adam's apple	the hard lump below the chin where the voice is made.
Adolescent	[A-dol-ES-nt] a young person between childhood and adulthood.
Afterbirth	see placenta.
Alcohol	[AL-ker-HOL] drink that effects the brain and body.
Amphetamine	[AM-fet-er-MEEN] addictive drug that speeds up the mind and body.
Anaemia	disease of weak blood. Signs are tiredness, pale gums and eyelids and no energy.
Anal intercourse	sexual intercourse into the anus.
Ante-natal	the months before a birth.
Antibiotic	medicine that fights infections.
Antibodies	special body chemicals in the blood which help fight disease.
Antiseptic	substance that destroys germs.
Anus	hole in man or woman where faeces come out.
Areola	[a-REE-ohla] dark area around the nipple on a breast.
Artificial insemination	conception in a woman without sexual intercourse, using semen put into her.
Aspirin	tablets which help headaches, fever and body pains. Can be bought in most shops. Can cause internal bleeding. Not suitable for children.
Backstreet abortion	illegal abortion.
Bacteria	[BAK-tear-rya] germs that cause many diseases.
Bag of waters	the bag inside the uterus that holds the water and the baby.
Balanced diet	eating a mixture of good food.
Barbiturate	[BAR-beet-YOO-rait] addictive sedative drug.
Barrier method	contraceptives that prevent sperm and ovum meeting. e.g. sheath, diaphragm.
Blackhead	small plug of dirt blocking a pore in the skin of the face, neck or back.

166

Blood transfusion	replacement of blood into body from another person.
Bilharzia	infectious disease caught from rivers.
Birth control	prevention of pregnancy.
Bisexual	someone who can physically love a man or a woman.
Bladder	the bag in the abdomen which holds urine.
Blood pressure	the pressure on the blood as it is pumped through the body.
Breakthrough bleeding	any unexpected bleeding between periods when a woman is taking The Pill. If frequent, change the type of Pill.
Breastfeeding	feeding a baby with mother's milk.
Breech birth	baby is born feet first.
Bronchitis	disease of the lungs. Signs of bronchitis are fever, coughing and pain in lungs.
Buttocks	part of the body that a person sits on.
Caesarian operation	[see-ZAIR-ree-yun] birth by operation through the abdomen.
Cancer	[KAN-sa] an abnormal growth in the body that can lead to death.
Cannabis	[KAN-ner-BEES] plant that is smoked that affects the brain.
Carbon monoxide	poisonous gas given off by tobacco smoke and motor exhaust.
Castration	[kas-TRAI-shn] removal by accident or operation of the testicles.
Cells	smallest unit of the body.
Centigrade	measure of temperature. Normal body temperature is 37°C. Water freezes at 0°C and boils at 100°C.
Cervix	[SER-viks] the opening or neck of the uterus at the top of the vagina.
Chancroid	[CHAN-kroid] a sexually transmitted disease
Child spacing	having a few years between each child in a family.
Chromosome	microscopic part of a body's cell that carries the genes.
Circulation	the flow of blood through the body.
Circumcision	[SUR-km-SEE-shn] operation to remove the foreskin.
Climax	see orgasm.
Clitoris	[KLEE-toh-rees] part of woman's vulva.
Cocaine	[KOA-kain] addictive drug that affects the brain.
Coil	an Intra-Uterine Device. Small piece of plastic fitted in a woman's uterus to prevent pregnancy.
Coitus	[KOH-ee-tus] joining together, or intercourse.
Coma	[KOA-mer] unconsciousness from which a person cannot be woken.
Combined Pill	contraceptive pill containing two hormones.
Complexion	[kom-PLEK-shn] condition of the skin.
Conception	[kon-SEP-shn] when the ovum and sperm join together and start to grow inside the woman.
Condom	[KON-dm] narrow plastic bag which fits over the man's penis to prevent pregnancy.
Constipation	[KON-stee-PAY-shn] difficulty in defaecating.
Consummation	[kon-SOO-maishun] the completion of marriage by sexual intercourse.

Contagious	[kontaijs] when a disease can be easily spread.
Contraception	[KON-tru-SEP-shn] any means used to prevent pregnancy.
Contraceptive	device or method of preventing pregnancy.
Contraction	[kon-TRAK-shn] tightening of the muscles, usually during birth.
Crabs	see pubic lice.
Cyst	[SEEst] unusual swelling containing fluid.
Cystitis	[sees-TI-tees] infection of the bladder. Signs are pain and need to urinate often.
Defaecate	[DEF-a-KAIT] discharge faeces from the body.
Deformed	not grown properly.
Dehydration	[DEE-hi-drai-SHUN] when the body lacks water.
Dentist	health worker who treats teeth.
Deodorant	body perfume.
Depo-Provera	brand name for one type of injectable contraceptive.
Diabetes	[DI-abeet-EES] disease affecting the blood and output of urine. Can be treated with a special diet and medicines.
Diaphragm	[DIE-er-FRAM] shallow plastic cap which fits over the cervix to prevent pregnancy.
Diarrhoea	[DYE-a-REE-ah] frequent runny or liquid faeces.
Disabled	handicapped, not able to do everything.
Discharge	loss of abnormal mucus or pus from the body.
Douche	[DOOSH] washing out the vagina with liquids.
Drug abuse	use of illegal drugs, which harm the body.
Durex	[dee-OO-rex] brand name for condom.
Ectopic	[ek-TO-peek] embryo growing in fallopian tubes. If left, an ectopic pregnancy can kill a woman.
Ejaculation	[ee-JAK-yoo-LAY-shn] release of semen from the penis at orgasm.
Embryo	[EM-bree-oh] unborn baby inside the uterus from conception up to 3 months, then it becomes a foetus.
Epididymis	[epee-DEE-dee-ms] long coiled tubes leading from testicles to vas, where sperm are formed.
Erection	[ee-REK-shn] when penis goes hard during sexual excitement.
Erogenous zones	[ee-ROJ-nus] areas of a man or woman's body which are most sensitive to sexual touch e.g. women: breasts, vulva, clitoris, mouth, behind ears, back of neck; men:mouth, nipples, penis, scrotum.
Faeces	[FEE-seez] solid waste which leaves the body through the anus. Stools; shit.
Fallopian tubes	[fal-LOh-pee-yan] two narrow tubes leading from the ovary to the uterus.
Family planning	using contraceptives to control pregnancy. See child spacing.
Fantasy	[FAN-ta-ZEE] imagined day dreams.
Feminine	behaving and looking like a woman.

Fertilization	[fer-TEE-lye-SAY-shn] joining of sperm and ovum.
Fertile days	days when a woman can become pregnant.
Fever	body temperature higher than normal.
Fibre	important part of food that prevents constipation. Found in fruit, vegetables and unrefined grains.
Foam	contraceptive used by woman.
Foetus	[FEE-tus] unborn baby from three months pregnancy to birth.
Foreskin	skin on end of penis.
Frigid	not enjoying sex.
Gay	homosexual.
Gender	[JEN-da] male or female.
Genes	[JEENz] part of human cells that influence growth and character.
Genital herpes	herpes of the genitals.
Genitals	[JE-neetls] external sexual parts; a man's penis and scrotum, a woman's vagina and vulva.
Glans	end of the penis.
Gonorrhoea	[GON-a-REE-ya] a sexually transmitted disease. First signs may be itching or sore genitals, discharge or may be no symptoms.
Groin	the front part of the body where the legs join.
Haemorrhage	heavy bleeding.
Hallucination	[hal-OOS-een-AI-shun] frightening thoughts and dreams, can be caused by drug abuse.
Hangover	effects of drinking too much alcohol-headache, body ache, vomiting, diarrhoea.
Hepatitis	disease of the liver, causes yellow eyes and black urine.
Hermaphrodite	[her-MAF-roh-dit] a person of both sexes (very rare).
Hernia	bulging of the intestines under abdomen skin.
Heroine	[HE-roa-EEN] illegal addictive drug, usually injected.
Herpes	[hir-PEEZ] disease of the mouth or genitals.
Heterosexual	someone who is sexually attracted to the opposite sex.
Homosexual	[HOM-oh-SEK-syool] a man or woman who is sexually attracted to the same sex.
Hormones	[HOR-mohnz] chemical messengers carried in the blood which cause changes in the body. Sex hormones are made in the testicles or the ovaries. When sex hormones are made children begin puberty.
Hot flush	hot burning felt by some women during menopause.
Hygiene	[HY-jeen] keeping clean.
Hymen	[HI-mn] soft skin partly covering vagina.
Hypertension	[HI-pa-TEN-shn] high blood pressure.
Immunity	[ee-MYOO-nee-TEE] an ability to fight off certain diseases.
Implant	contraceptive device placed under woman's skin.
Impotence	inability of man to have erection.

Incest sex between brothers and sisters or parents and their children.

Infection [een-FEK-shn] disease caused by germs, which may affect part of the body, (such as infected finger), or the whole body, (such as gonorrhoea).

Infertile unable to conceive, see sterile.

Inflammation [EEN-fla-MAI-shn] redness and swelling with infection.

Injectable contraceptive injected into woman.

Injection [een-JEK-shn] medicine given to person into skin through a needle.

Intra-Uterine Device, small piece of plastic fitted into the uterus to prevent pregnancy.
or IUD Also called the Coil or Loop.

Jab, The injectable contraceptive.

Junk food food that does not help the body, and may harm it. Sweets, cool drinks, hamburgers, alcohol.

Kidneys [KEED-neez] two organs in abdomen where urine is filtered.

Labia [LAY-bee-ya] lips of the vulva.

Labour contractions of the uterus before birth of a baby.

Larynx [LA-ree-nks] tube in neck where voice is made.

Lesbian woman who is sexually attracted to other women.

Libido enjoyment of sex.

Liver part of the body which absorbs and stores nutrients from food, and manufactures many important body chemicals.

Loop see Intra-Uterine Device.

Lubricant oil, jelly or cream to make surfaces slippery.

LSD illegal drug that affects the brain.

Lust sexual desire.

Malaria disease caught from mosquitoes.

Masai tribe in East Africa of very tall people.

Masculine looking and behaving like a man.

Masturbation [MAS-tur-BAI-shun] sexually arousing oneself.

Menarche [MEN-ark] the time when girls start having periods, usually between 10 and 16 years.

Menopause the time when a woman stops having periods, usually between 45 and 55 years.

Menses see menstruation.

Menstrual cycle [MEN-stroo-ul] the changes every month in a woman's body relating to reproduction-periods, ovulation, hormone changes.

Menstruation [MEN-stroo-AI-shn] the few days each month that a woman's uterus bleeds.

Menstrual period see menstruation.

Microscope an instrument that makes very small objects look larger.

Midwife woman who helps a mother during labour and birth.

Mini-Pill	contraceptive pill with small dose of one hormone.
Mini-towel	small paper pad for periods.
Miraa	poisonous plant chewed to reduce fatigue and hunger.
Miscarriage	pregnancy ending before 6 months; death of foetus.
Monogamy	being married to one partner.
Morning sickness	nausea and vomiting in the morning during pregnancy.
Morphine	[MOR-f-EEN] addictive painkilling drug which affects the brain.
Mucus	[MYOO-cus] slippery clear liquid produced by wet parts of the body.
Nausea	[NOR-see-ya] feeling one wants to vomit.
Navel	[NAI-vul] scar in middle of abdomen where umbilical cord was attached before birth.
Nicotine	poisonous chemical in cigarettes and tobacco.
Non-specific	cause not exactly known.
Nutritious	foods that help the body grow, be healthy and fight disease.
Opium	[OH-pee-YUM] addictive illegal drug made from poppy plant.
Oral contraceptive	contraceptive pill swallowed every day.
Oral sex	sexual actitivy where the mouth or tongue is applied to the sex organs of the partner.
Orgasm	climax of pleasant physical and emotional feelings during sexual intercourse. In men this includes ejaculation and muscle contractions around the genitals. In women orgasms include a warm glow or buzz around the genitals, or all over the body.
Ovaries	[OH-varee] two organs inside a woman where sex hormones and ovum are made.
Overdose	taking too much drug or medicine and causing harm to the body, or death.
Ovulation	[OH-vyoo-LAI-shn] when the ovary releases an ovum each month.
Ovum	[OH-voom] egg produced by woman once a month.
Oxygen	[OK-see-jun] gas in the air that keeps people alive.
Paracetamol	[PA-rah-SEE-to-MOL] medicine which helps aches, pains and fevers. Safer then aspirin for children, and adults.
Paralysis	[per-RAL-ee-SEES] loss of movement in part of body.
Pelvic infection	infection in the lower abdomen of a woman, involving her reproductive organs.
Pelvis	[PEL-vees] lower part of the abdomen, including internal sexual organs.
Penis	[PEE-nees] male sex organ.
Perineum	[PE-ra-NEE-yum] muscle between woman's anus and vagina.
Periods	monthly bleeding from the uterus in a woman.
Pessary	medicine or contraceptive placed in vagina.
Petroleum jelly	thick white cream used on face and hair. Brand name: Vaseline.
Petting	kissing, stroking, touching a lover.

Pharmacy	shop that sells medicines.
Pill, The	tablet taken by women to prevent pregnancy.
Placenta	[pla-SEN-ta] part in the uterus which filters the blood going from the mother to the foetus.
Platonic	[pla-TON-eek] non physical love.
Pneumonia	[noo-MOH-nya] disease of the lungs. Causes fever, pain and sometimes death if not treated.
Polygamy	[po-LEE-ger-MEE] having more than one wife or husband.
Pores	the small holes in the skin, where acne appears.
Post-coital	after sexual intercourse.
Pregnancy	time when woman is expecting a baby.
Premature birth	baby born before 38 weeks pregnancy.
Pre-menstrual tension	or PMT-depression, tiredness or irritability a few days before a woman's period.
Prepuce	foreskin.
Prostate	gland-a small bag at the base of a man's bladder.
Prostitute	woman who makes money from sex.
Pubic hair	[PYOO-beek] hair growing around the genitals.
Pubic lice	tiny insects living in pubic hair.
Puberty	[PYOO-bertee] age when children start developing into adults.
Pus	yellow or white liquid from infected parts of the body. Pus is full of bacteria.
Pygmy	tribe in Central Africa of very small people.
Rape	sexual intercourse without woman's consent.
Resistant disease	a disease that cannot be cured with drugs.
Rhythm method	natural method of contraception without using drugs or devices.
Ringworm	mild disease of the skin. More common among people who do not wash. Treated with special cream.
Rubella	[roo-BEL-a] mild disease that can cause deformity in baby if mother catches rubella during early pregnancy. Also called German Measles.
Sanitary towel	pad of cotton-wool used by women during their periods.
Scabies	skin disease caused by small insects. Easily treated with medicine.
Scrotum	[sk-ROH-tm] the bag behind the man's penis which holds the testicles.
Sebaceous glands	[ser-BAI-shus] tiny sacs inside the skin where natural skin oil is produced.
Secondary sexual characteristics	pubic hair, breasts, beard.
Sedative	any drug that slows down the body and brain.
Semen	[SEE-men] white fluid produced by man which carries the sperm through his penis into the woman's uterus.
Sex	1) Either male or female. 2) Shortened word for sexual intercourse.

Sex maniac	a man who is obsessed with sex and may want to rape women.
Sexual intercourse	the act of making love where the penis is placed inside the vagina.
Sexually transmitted disease	disease that is caught from sexual partners. STDs include gonorrhoea, syphilis, AIDS, herpes.
Sheath	same as condom.
Shot, The	injectable contraceptive.
Sickle cell anaemia	disorder in the blood inherited from parents.
Side-effects	problems in the body after taking medicines or drugs.
Skull	bones of the head.
Smear test	medical test for cancer of the cervix.
Smegma	[s-MEG-ma] sticky secretion on a man's glans.
Sperm	male eggs.
Spermicide	[sPER-mee-SA-yeed] chemical which kills sperm. Used with diaphragms and sheaths as contraception.
Sponge, The	sponge inserted into vagina during intercourse to prevent pregnancy.
Spontaneous abortion	see miscarriage.
Sterile	unable to conceive, infertile. Or completely germ free.
Sterilization	operation for a man or woman to prevent pregnancy permanently.
Stethoscope	medical instrument for listening to heart beat and breathing.
Suction evacuation	method of abortion.
Symptoms	[SEEM-ptms] signs of a disease or illness. For example, headache or fever.
Syphilis	[SEE-fee-lees] sexually transmitted disease. If not treated can lead to disability or death.
Syringe	[SEE-REE-nj] instrument with a sharp needle for injecting medicines.
Taboo	an act or subject which is avoided or not permitted in a society.
Tampon	cotton-wool placed in vagina during period.
Testicle	[TES-tee-kul] the two small organs in a man's scrotum where sperm and sex hormones are produced.
Tetanus	disease from infected wounds, often leading to death.
Thermometer	instrument for measuring the temperature of the body.
Thrush	infection in the mouth or a woman's vagina.
Transmitted	passed on to someone else.
Triplets	three babies born together.
Twins	two babies born together.
Umbilical cord	[um-BEE-lee-kl] the tube carrying blood to the foetus from the placenta.
Unconscious	when someone appears to be asleep, but cannot be woken up. Usually after an accident to the head, or an overdose of drugs or alcohol.

Urethra [yoo-REE-thra] tube which carries urine from the bladder to the penis or vulva.

Urethritis [YOO-ree-THRY-tus] infection of the urethra.

Urine [YOO-reen] liquid waste from body.

Urinary infection [YOO-ree-nay-ree] infection of the urethra, bladder or kidneys.

Uterus [YOO-tu-rus] bag of muscle where unborn baby develops inside the mother. Also called womb.

Vagina [vaj-EYE-na] tube leading from vulva to the uterus in a woman.

Varicose veins [VA-reek-OHZ] abnormal swelling of the leg veins.

Vas narrow tube leading from testicles to penis.

Vasectomy [vas-EK-toh-mee] operation on a man to cut vas to prevent pregnancy in his wife.

Veneral disease see sexually transmitted disease.

Virgin [VER-jeen] male or female who has not had sexual intercourse.

Virile [VEE-ra-eel] man with strong sexual characteristics.

Vitamins protective foods our bodies need to work properly.

Vulva [VUL-va] woman's external genitals.

Warts small, rough bumps on the skin.

Wet dreams sexual dreams of a man, with ejaculation while asleep.

Withdrawal method of contraception by taking penis out of vagina before ejaculating.

Womb [WOOM] see uterus.

References

Bell, R., *Changing Bodies, Changing Lives, A Book for Teens on Sex and Relationships*, Random House, 1980.

Centre for African Family Studies, *An Introduction to Family Life Education in Africa*, Kenya, no date.
Centre for African Family Studies, *Family Life Education Curriculum Guidelines*, Kenya, 1984.
Center for Disease Control, *Family Planning Methods and Practice in Africa*, USA, 1983.
Clarity Collective, *Taught Not Caught*, Learning Development Aids, UK, 1983.
Cousins, J., *Make It Happy*, Virago, 1978.

Dean, P., *Talks to Teenagers*, unpublished, 1979.
Docharty, J., *Growing Up*, Alcamco, Nigeria, 1982.
Durex Contraception Information Service, *Sex and Health*, 1984.

Guillebaud, J., *The Pill*, Oxford University Press, 1984.
Guillebaud, J., *Contraception. Your Questions Answered*, Churchill Livingstone, 1986.

Hampton, J., *Happy Healthy Children*, Macmillan, 1985.
Health Education Council, *Pregnancy Book*, UK, 1984.
Health Education Council, *Guide to a Healthy Sex Life*, 1985.

International Childrens Centre, *Education on Sexuality, the Family and Society Today*, Children in the Tropics, France, 1985.
International Planned Parenthood Federation, *Introducing Contraception*, UK, 1979.

Kleinman, R., *Adolescent Sex, its difficulties and dangers*, International Planned Parenthood Federation, 1978.

Lee, C., *The Ostrich Position*, Writers and Readers, 1983.

Mayle, P., and Robins, A., *We're Not Pregnant*, Macmillan, 1981.

Meredith, S., *Growing Up*, Usborne, 1985.

Phillips, A., and Rakusen, J., *Our Bodies, Ourselves*, Penguin, UK, 1978.

Plain English Campaign, *Drug Alert*, BBC Broadcasting Support Services, UK, 1985.

Terence Higgins Trust, *A.I.D.S., The Facts*, 1986.

Thomson, R., *Have You Started Yet?*, Heinemann, 1980.

Went, D., *Sex Education, some guidelines for teachers*, Bell & Hyman, 1985.

Werner, D., *Where There Is No Doctor*, Macmillan, 1978.

Index

umbilical cord, 52, 65
urethra, 19
urethritis, 127—8
urination, 61
urine, 'burning', 124, 126, 127—8
uterus, 21, 53—4, 65
  infection, 89

VD, see STD
vagina, 20
  dry, 5, 25
  infection of, 32, 127, 145—6
  itchy, 127
vas, 30, 104
vasectomy, 104—7
venereal disease, see STD
virginity, 42

voice, change in, 26
vomiting, 61, 83
vulva, 19

warts, genital, 125
washing, 137, 138
water, in uterus, 53, 63, 64
weight increase, 158
wet dreams, 44—5
woman, 'ideal', 14—15
womb, see uterus
work
  and alcohol, 152
  after birth, 65
  and marriage, 8

yeast infection, 128

UNIVERSITY of WOLVERHAMPTON